Fundamental Mathematics
for Epidemiology Study

RAY M. MERRILL, PhD, MPH

Brigham Young University
Provo, Utah

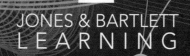

JONES & BARTLETT
LEARNING

World Headquarters
Jones & Bartlett Learning
5 Wall Street
Burlington, MA 01803
978-443-5000
info@jblearning.com
www.jblearning.com

Jones & Bartlett Learning books and products are available through most bookstores and online booksellers. To contact Jones & Bartlett Learning directly, call 800-832-0034, fax 978-443-8000, or visit our website, www.jblearning.com.

Substantial discounts on bulk quantities of Jones & Bartlett Learning publications are available to corporations, professional associations, and other qualified organizations. For details and specific discount information, contact the special sales department at Jones & Bartlett Learning via the above contact information or send an email to specialsales@jblearning.com.

12740-9

Production Credits
VP, Product Management: David D. Cella
Director of Product Management: Michael Brown
Product Specialist: Carter McAlister
Associate Production Editor: Alex Schab
Senior Marketing Manager: Sophie Fleck Teague
Production Services Manager: Colleen Lamy
Manufacturing and Inventory Control Supervisor: Amy Bacus
Composition: codeMantra U.S. LLC
Cover Design: Kristin E. Parker
Text Design: Kristin E. Parker
Director of Rights & Media: Joanna Gallant
Rights & Media Specialist: Merideth Tumasz
Media Development Editor: Shannon Sheehan
Cover Image (Title Page, Chapter Opener):
    © Nongkran_ch/Getty Images
Printing and Binding: LSC Communications
Cover Printing: LSC Communications

Library of Congress Cataloging-in-Publication Data
Names: Merrill, Ray M., author.
Title: Fundamental mathematics for epidemiology study / Ray M. Merrill.
Description: Burlington, Massachusetts: Jones & Bartlett Learning, 2018.
Identifiers: LCCN 2018015407 | ISBN 9781284127331 (paperback)
Subjects: LCSH: Epidemiology—Mathematical models. | BISAC: EDUCATION / General.
Classification: LCC RA652.2.M3 M462 2018 | DDC 614.401/5118—dc23
LC record available at https://lccn.loc.gov/2018015407

6048

Printed in the United States of America
22 21 20 19 18   10 9 8 7 6 5 4 3 2 1

To Gerald and Janice

Contents

About the Author

Ray M. Merrill received his academic training in statistics and public health. In 1995, he was a Cancer Prevention Fellow at the National Cancer Institute, where he was able to apply his quantitative training to the field of cancer epidemiology. In 1998, he joined the faculty in the Department of Health Science at Brigham Young University in Provo, Utah, where he has been active in teaching and research. In 2001, he spent a sabbatical working in the Unit of Epidemiology for Cancer Prevention at the International Agency for Research on Cancer Administration in Lyon, France. Dr. Merrill has won various awards for his research and is a Fellow of the American College of Epidemiology and of the American Academy of Health Behavior. He is the author of more than 250 peer-reviewed publications, including *Environmental Epidemiology, Reproductive Epidemiology, Principles of Epidemiology Workbook, Fundamentals of Epidemiology and Biostatistics, Behavioral Epidemiology,* and *Statistical Methods in Epidemiologic Research* (all published by Jones & Bartlett Learning). Dr. Merrill is a professor at Brigham Young University, teaching courses in epidemiology and biostatistics for the Department of Health Science within the College of Life Sciences.

Preface

Mathematical concepts and their applications are central to epidemiology. Mathematics provides an approach used in epidemiology to describe and analyze health-related states or events. Descriptive epidemiology involves describing the distribution (frequency and pattern) of health-related states or events. This often concerns determining the number of events and often presenting the number of events as a rate. The number or rate of a health event may be presented according to person, place, and time factors, thereby helping us see how these characteristics are associated with the health problem. Numbers are arithmetic values that are used to identify the extent of a public health problem and, when expressed as a rate, can reflect risk.

The primary subdivisions of mathematics are arithmetic, algebra, geometry, and calculus. Statistics is a branch of mathematics that deals with collecting, analyzing, interpreting, and presenting numerical data. Analytic epidemiology aims to identify causes of health-related states or events. Identifying a statistical association between variables can help support the possibility of a causal relationship. If a causal association is present, a statistical association exists, although the converse is not necessarily true.

This book has three main purposes:

1. Present fundamental math principles and procedures used in epidemiology
2. Identify the math principles and procedures that are appropriate for specific epidemiologic study designs
3. Apply Excel and Epi Info™ 7 to assess selected epidemiologic data

This is an introductory textbook aimed at providing

- Data visualization tools
- Digitally interactive learning progression
- Instructions on how to apply Excel and Epi Info™ 7 (freeware downloadable from the Centers for Disease Control and Prevention [CDC] website) to describe and assess health problems

Along with this book, the author provides computer application problems, as well as practice problems that can be solved online, with instant feedback and a review of corresponding concepts. Chapter problems evaluate mastery of selected learning outcomes that involve basic math principles and procedures:

1. Remembering—recognizing and recalling relevant mathematical concepts
2. Understanding—interpreting and explaining mathematical summary measures, charts, graphs, and tables
3. Applying—generating, or testing specific hypotheses, performing statistical tests, and computing and charting age-adjusted rates and other epidemiologic health indicators for given study designs

4. Analyze—identifying stages of disease progression and comparing health outcomes according to exposure classifications

5. Evaluate—monitoring and testing for the internal and external consistency of selected study designs

A study's level of *internal* consistency has to do with the extent to which its results are true for the target population. A study's level of *external* consistency has to do with the extent to which its results are appropriately generalized to other populations. Evaluation also involves making judgements based on criteria and standards (e.g., causal guidelines), as will be developed in more advanced epidemiology texts.

Mastery of these learning outcomes will prepare the student for more advanced training and application in the field of epidemiology. Along the way, skills will be learned for effectively assessing and monitoring the health of populations at risk and identifying health problems and priorities. Additionally, the ability to identify risk factors for health problems and to predict the effects of certain exposures and interventions will also be taught. These skills, in turn, can help formulate policies and priorities designed to solve identified health problems and allocate scarce health resources for preventing, protecting, and promoting the public's health.

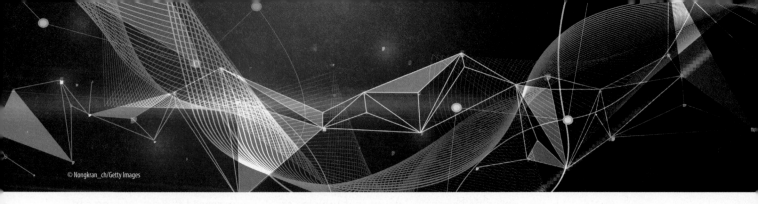

CHAPTER 1

Mathematics in Epidemiology

Mathematics is the study of numbers, equations, shapes, and relationships. It is a deterministic way of viewing our quantitative world. Its primary subdivisions are arithmetic, algebra, geometry, and calculus. Statistics is a branch of mathematics that deals with collecting, analyzing, interpreting, and presenting numerical data. As such, it is useful for describing data and drawing conclusions about characteristics in the population based on sample data.

The purpose of this chapter is to describe the history of modern epidemiology and the important role this discipline plays in public health. The general use of mathematics in epidemiology will be explored.

▶ Applying Math in Epidemiology

Since the middle part of the 20th century, there has been a proliferation of epidemiologic studies. These studies have been successful at describing many health states and events and in identifying attributes, characteristics, or exposures associated with increased risk for several diseases or injuries (**risk factors**). For example, we now know many of the primary explanations for cancer: 29–31% tobacco, 20–50% diet, 10–20% infections (bacteria, viruses), 5–7% ionizing and UV light, 2–4% occupation, and 1–5% pollution (air, water, food).[1] A greater availability of disease and health-related data helps explain much of the rapid increase in epidemiologic studies. In the United States, Europe, and elsewhere we currently have several large surveys and data collection systems that are regularly conducted (e.g., the National Health Interview Survey, the Behavior Risk Factor Surveillance System, the National Health and Nutrition Examination Survey, the National Health Care Surveys, the European Network of Cancer Registries, and GLOBOCAN). Routine collection of vital statistics and widespread use of research questionnaires and experimental research have further contributed to the rapid increase of data.

As the discipline has matured, epidemiology has increasingly drawn upon numbers and their operations to describe disease and health-related states and conditions. Several individuals with mathematical training have contributed in important ways to epidemiology. For example, Florence Nightingale (1820–1910) applied mathematical analysis to measure social phenomena and determine the average time required to transport patients for medical care.[2] Wade Hampton Frost (1880–1938) provided the first mathematical expression of the epidemic curve.[3] In 1956, a prospective cohort study of British doctors provided statistical proof that tobacco smoking increased the risk of lung cancer.[4] Beginning in the 1960s, Olli S. Miettinen (1936–) developed and promoted several statistical and causal approaches to epidemiology in a series of landmark papers;[5-8] Jerome Cornfield (1912–1979) helped develop clinical trials, Bayesian inference, and the relationship between statistical theory and practice;[9] Joseph L. Fleiss (1937–2003) contributed to mental health research by developing statistical measures of inter-rater reliability;[10,11] Norman Breslow (1941–2015) developed and promoted the case-control matched sample design and advanced ways to calculate survival rates for disease;[12] and William G. Cochran (1909–1980) developed and advanced experimental designs and sampling techniques.[14-16] In 1982, Kleinbaum, Kupper, and Morgenstern contributed to epidemiology with the first comprehensive book to describe objectives and methods of epidemiologic research, the validity of epidemiologic research, and principles and procedures of epidemiologic analysis.[17] These are just a few of the many individuals who have built upon a mathematical foundation to advance the field of epidemiology.

▶ The Role of Epidemiology in Public Health

Public health is a social institution, a practice and service concerned with safeguarding and improving the health of individuals on the community level. **Epidemiology** is the part of public health that focuses on individuals who share one or more observable characteristics from which data can be collected and analyzed. It is the study of the **distribution** (frequency and pattern) and **determinants** of disease (e.g., congenital and hereditary, allergies and inflammatory, degenerative, metabolic, cancer), events (e.g., injury, accident, drug overdose, suicide), behaviors (e.g., physical activity, diet, safety precautions), and existing conditions (e.g., a state of fitness, an unhealthy state). It includes the application of this study to prevent and control diseases and other health-related problems. Epidemiology provides an approach to assess and monitor the health status of populations and to identify health problems and priorities, risk factors for disease, and valuable health interventions; it also provides an approach to predict the influence on health of an infectious or toxic chemical agent, an individual attribute (e.g., age, race/ethnicity, gender), or a behavior (e.g., physical activity, tobacco use, weight management). Epidemiologic information, in turn, can inform and motivate individuals to avoid certain exposures, adopt important health behaviors, and promote more effective public health planning, communication, decision-making, and implementation of interventions.

The study of the distribution of health-related states or events involves surveillance and descriptive methods. **Descriptive methods** are used to monitor health status and environmental hazards, establish whether a health problem exists, identify those at greatest risk, and reveal when and where the health problem is greatest.

The study of the determinants of health-related states or events combines analytic methods and causal theory. **Analytic methods** explore whether a given exposure is associated with a disease or other health-related outcome. The exposure may be related to the environment (e.g., radon gas, chemical pollution, air pollution), lifestyle (e.g., lack of physical activity, unhealthy diet, smoking), condition (e.g., high blood cholesterol, high blood pressure, stress), or inherent characteristics (e.g., fair skin, mutation in one of the BRCA genes, immediate relative has type 1 diabetes). An **exposure** may be a specific event and relatively easy to measure, or it may be indirect and require proxy measures or estimates obtained through modeling. Causal guidelines (e.g., valid statistical association, temporal sequence of events, biologic plausibility) have been proposed to support deterministic relationships and to provide an understanding of the mechanisms that underlie the problem. Both descriptive and analytic epidemiologic information contribute to preventing and controlling health problems such as diseases.

Overall, epidemiology combines elements of medicine, sociology, demography, and mathematics. Epidemiologists use math operations when tracking the progress of infectious disease, identifying the success rates of interventions, communicating health findings, and much more. Mathematical models are used to track the transmission, spread, and control of infectious disease; the virulence of disease; and the persistence of pathogens in their hosts. They also help us better understand the underlying mechanisms that influence the spread of disease.

▶ Numbers in Epidemiology

Epidemiology has a scientific basis that relies heavily on a systematic and unbiased approach of data collection, analysis, and interpretation. **Data** is information obtained through observation, experiment, or measurement of a phenomenon of interest; it consists of facts like numbers, words, observations, measurements, or descriptions. Numerical data is obtained from variables. A **variable** is a condition, factor, or trait that varies from one observation to the next, may be measured or categorized, and can take on a specified set of values. It represents a number we do not know yet, as opposed to a fixed number.

Numbers are arithmetic values used in counting, making calculations, identifying subjects, and showing the position in a series. Epidemiologists characterize public health problems by identifying the number of new cases of a health-related state or event in a given time period (incidence), deaths in a given time period (mortality), and the number of existing cases up to a point in time (prevalence). These measures are often made more meaningful by expressing them in terms of their originating population. Specifically, the number of cases occurring during a specified time period is divided by the population at risk during the same time period to obtain an incidence rate; the number of deaths occurring during a specified time period is divided by the population from which the deaths occurred to obtain a mortality rate; and the number of all existing cases is divided by the population at a given time to obtain a point prevalence proportion. Presenting these measures according to person, place, and time factors can provide additional information that is useful for understanding, preventing, and controlling health problems.

In the context of data collection and management, members of a study population may be assigned a unique identifying number (called a **sampling frame**), which is required for probabilistic sampling, data linkage, and confidentiality.

A number may also be used to show the position in a series, such as indicating the level of preference, with one end of a scale labeled as the most positive and the other end labeled as the most negative. In a graphic rating scale (continuous rating scale), the ends of the continuum are typically labeled with opposite values. The **Likert scale** generally involves an odd number of choices (usually 1–5 or 7), ranging from least to most.

▶ Equations in Epidemiology

An **equation** is a statement that indicates that the values of two mathematical expressions are equal. For example, the following equation says the difference in two population means is equal to 5: $\mu_1 - \mu_2 = 5$. A **formula** is a special type of equation, frequently used in epidemiology, that shows the relationship between different variables. The prevalence of a health-related state or event is directly influenced by incidence and duration; prevalence = incidence × average duration (survival, cure). As incidence increases, then prevalence increases. For example, as survival increases, average duration and prevalence increase. As people are cured, average duration and prevalence decrease.

The formula used to convey disease risk is:

$$\text{Attack rate} = \text{Cumulative incidence rate} = \frac{\text{Number of disease cases}}{\text{Size of the population initially at risk}}$$

For example, suppose that 50 people ate a contaminated food and 40 became ill. The attack rate is 80 per 100, or 80%.

If the denominator is the sum of person-time rather than the number of people, then we call it a "rate" and the formula is:

$$\text{Person-time rate} = \text{Incidence density rate} = \frac{\text{Number of disease cases}}{\text{Sum of person-time}}$$

For example, suppose there were 10 injuries that occurred at a company in 4 weeks. The time on the job differed among the employees, with 80 working 40 hours per week, 25 working 20 hours per week, and 10 working 50 hours per week.

The total hours worked for these employees is

$$4 \times (80 \times 40 + 25 \times 20 + 10 \times 50) = 4 \times 4,200 = 16,800$$

Then, the rate is

$$\frac{10}{16,800} = 0.000595$$

To improve the interpretation of the rate, we can multiply by 100,000 and round up, giving 60 injuries per 100,000 hours worked.

The formula for measuring prevalence proportion is:

$$\text{Prevalence proportion} = \frac{\text{Number of existing cases on a specific date}}{\text{Number of people in the population on this date}}$$

For example, suppose 45 adults who completed a questionnaire indicated that they currently smoke cigarettes. If 500 people completed the questionnaire, then the prevalence proportion is

$$\frac{45}{500} = 0.09$$

We can multiply this value by 100 to produce a more interpretable result: 9 per 100 or 9%.

Other formulas commonly used in epidemiology will be presented in later chapters.

▶ Patterns and Shapes Used in Epidemiology

To depict important patterns of health-related states or events in the population, counts or rates of the health events are often presented according to person (who), place (where), and time (when) variables. Identifying who is at greatest risk and gaining causal insights can result in identifying who is being affected, where the problem is most common, and when the problem has the greatest chance of occurring. In other words, the reason certain health-related states or events occur among some people but not others, in some places but not others, and at some times but not others, provides insight into what may be causing the health problem.

Person characteristics include inherent traits (e.g., age, gender, race/ethnicity), activities (e.g., occupation, leisure, use of medications, education, marriage family), and conditions (e.g., access to health care, clean water, good housing conditions; sanitation). **Place** involves identifying the concentration of cases by areas such as residence, birthplace, place of employment, school district, hospital unit, country, county, census tract, street address, map coordinates, and so on. **Time** aspects are chronological events, step-by-step occurrences, chains of events tied to time, and the time distribution of the onset of cases.

Person

"Person" data is usually displayed in tables and graphs. The most commonly assessed person characteristics are age and sex. Most health-related states or events vary by age. Age is associated with disease susceptibility, physiological response, incubation periods, and opportunity for exposure. Most disease and death rates are higher for males. Inherent differences between males and females (e.g., hormonal, genetic, anatomic) influence physiologic responses. Differences in occupation, lifestyle, and risk behaviors also explain differences in susceptibility. For example, "person" variables like poverty, low education, lack of work skills, and disrupted families have each been shown to increase the risk of the top eight leading causes of death in the United States: heart disease, cancer, stroke, accidents, diabetes, cirrhosis, suicide, and homicide.[18]

Place

"Place" data of residence or any other geographic location relevant to the occurrence of the health problem is often presented using tables, graphs, and maps. Comparison of counts or rates of health-related states or events among communities allow us to identify higher risk groups. A community at greater risk may be explained by specific characteristics about the people (e.g., risk behaviors, exposure to local toxins or food contaminants, genetic susceptibility); an infectious agent (e.g., a vector, a virulent strain, a hospitable breeding environment); or an environmental factor that influences the risk of disease transmission from person to person (e.g., crowded urban spaces, homes built in areas near deer or larger animal populations that carry black-legged ticks with Lyme disease). The following graph provides an example of the rates of suicide among white males and females in the United States, 2012–2014 (**FIGURE 1.1**).

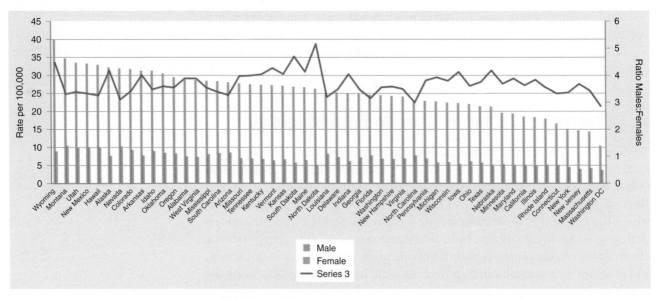

FIGURE 1.1 Suicide in the United States for whites, 2012–2014

Data from: Surveillance, Epidemiology, and End Results (SEER) Program (www.seer.cancer.gov) SEER*Stat Database: Mortality - All COD, Aggregated With State, Total U.S. (1969–2014) <Katrina/Rita Population Adjustment>, National Cancer Institute, DCCPS, Surveillance Research Program, released December 2016. Underlying mortality data provided by NCHS (www.cdc.gov/nchs).

The highest suicide rates tend to be in the western states, and the lowest tend to be in the eastern states. Suicide rates among males are 2.8 to 5.2 greater than for females.

Medical geography is an area of health research that studies how locale and climate influence health-related states or events. In geography, the term "location" describes a place with respect to residence (village, city, and town) and environment, whereas "place" describes the person and physical characteristics of a location. The idea that location and place may affect health is not new. Hippocrates (460–377 BC) understood that certain diseases were associated with place when he described malaria as more common in people who lived at lower elevations, near swampy areas.[19] These areas are where mosquitos breed and can convey disease through their bite.

A classic application of medical geography was performed by John Snow (1813–1858), a physician and anesthesiologist in England, who identified fecal-contaminated water as the source of a cholera epidemic in London.[20] He did this by plotting both water supplies and cholera deaths on a map and observing their relationship. Some health-related states or events that involve many cases over large geographic areas are presented on an area map. This type of map represents different levels of counts or rates by shades of color over geographic areas. For example, the Census Data Mapper is an interactive webapp where the percentage of selected demographic factors according to US counties can be identified.

In the past few decades, the **geographic information system (GIS)** has been increasingly used in medical geography. GIS is a computer technique that combines spatial information with one or more layers of attribute information. **Spatial data** describes location. There are four types of spatial data: (1) continuous (e.g., elevation, ultraviolet exposure, precipitation); (2) areas (unbounded: radon gas, forests, land use, bounded: city, county, state, and health boundaries, moving: mosquito areas, air masses, ozone gas); (3) networks (e.g., roads, rivers, power lines); and (4) points (fixed, such as wells, addresses, street lights or moving, such as cars, airplanes, animals). **Attribute data** specifies characteristics of that location (e.g., city names, type of road, temperature, rainfall, address). Medical GIS is commonly used to test statistically whether (1) clustering of health-related states or events exists in certain locations (i.e., non-random spatial distributions), (2) patterns of health problems associate with human behavior or environmental factors, and (3) there is adequate access or a need for additional healthcare services according to visual displays of population densities and income levels.[21]

Time

Outbreaks of disease are often described by graphing the number of cases by the time of onset of illness. An **epidemic curve** is a graph of the frequency or magnitude of disease across time, showing the course of the health problem. It identifies the most likely time of exposure and is used to formulate hypotheses about the type of disease involved and its mode of transmission. The time between exposure to a pathogen (i.e., virus, bacteria, fungus, and parasite), chemical, or radiation and the clinical manifestations of the disease is the **incubation period**. Because the incubation period for several major diseases is known, if our investigation identifies the incubation period for those exposed, we can get a good idea of the causal agent involved. For example, influenza has an incubation period of 1–3 days, with communicability typically 3 days from clinical onset.

Some epidemic curves show a rapid increase in the number of incident cases, a peak, and then a decline (**FIGURE 1.2**). The graph identifies where the distribution of data has its peak (central location), the dispersion of the data around the peak (spread), and whether the distribution of data is symmetric on both sides of the peak.

A single peaked distribution that is right skewed (positively skewed) has a long right tail. A distribution that is left skewed (negatively skewed) has a long left tail. Skewed data occurs when outlying cases that stand apart from the general distribution are present.

The shape of the frequency distribution will influence the measure of central tendency and dispersion. The mean is more sensitive to outliers than the median, and the median is more sensitive to outliers than the mode, as illustrated using data on deaths from a cholera outbreak in the Golden Square of London (**FIGURE 1.3**). In this figure, the mode is day 3, the median is day 9, and the mean is day 10.2.

A "propagated" (or "progressive source") epidemic involves an index case that infects other people, who subsequently become ill. The **index case** in an

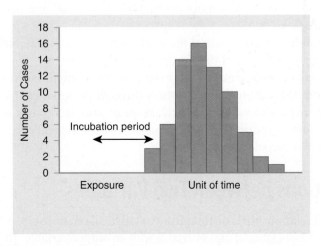

FIGURE 1.2 Epidemic curve: Point source

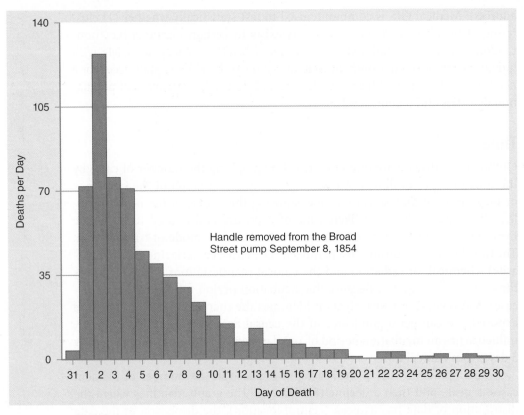

FIGURE 1.3 Cholera outbreak in the Golden Square of London, August 31–September 30, 1854

Data from Whitehad, H. Remarks on the outbreak of cholera in broad street, Golden Square, London, in 1954. *Transactions of the Epidemiological Society of London*, Vol. 3. Read at a meeting of the Society on 6 May 1867.

epidemiologic study is the first case to come to the attention of investigators. One or more of the infected people in this first wave of cases infects other people, who become ill. Propagated epidemics generally involve a series of successively larger peaks, which reflect the incubation period of the disease (e.g., an average of about 10 days for measles; **FIGURE 1.4**), until control measures are successfully implemented or there is no longer a pool of susceptible people.

Intermittent environmental exposures may lead to an epidemic curve involving a series of peaks separated by the average incubation period for the disease. A continuous source exposure (e.g., radiation) tends to result in illness reflected in the epidemic curve with a more gradual increase, peak, and decrease in the frequency of cases.

It is possible to have a mixed epidemic, which involves a combination of a point source outbreak and then propagation of the disease. For example, an initial outbreak of cholera may result from drinking contaminated water. Then, the cases from this outbreak infect others through personal contact. Thus, the epidemic curve may show a sharp increase, peak, and decrease of several cases, and then, following the disease incubation period, subsequent ebbs and flows in the number of infected cases.

▶ Relations between Two Variables

A functional relationship is distinct from a statistical relationship. A **functional relationship** associates an input variable with an output variable. The functional

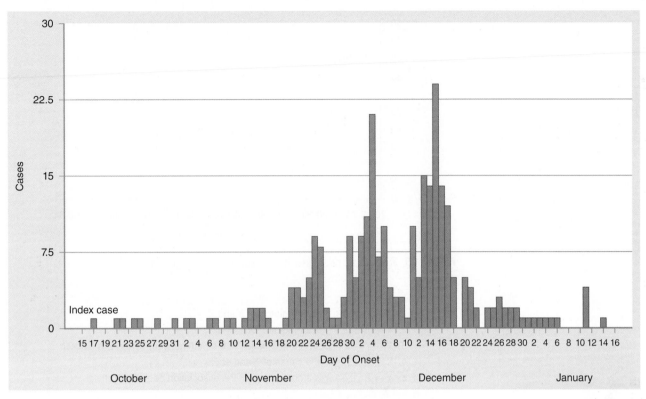

FIGURE 1.4 Measles cases by date of onset, October 15, 1970–January 16, 1971

Data from: Aberdeen, S.D. Centers for Disease Control and Prevention. Measles outbreak. MMWR, 1971;20:26.

relationship between an exposure variable x and a health outcome variable y is of the form

$$y = f(x)$$

For a given value of x, the function f gives the corresponding value of y. For example, suppose that five men die prematurely (prior to their retirement age at 65 years) because of a worksite accident. Their ages are 27, 34, 55, 25, and 60. The association between their ages and years of potential life lost (YPLL) through retirement at age 65 is

$$y = f(x) = 65 - x$$

The YPLL for each person is shown in the right column of the following table.

Person	Age	YPLL
1	27	38
2	34	31
3	55	10
4	25	40
5	60	5

The total YPLL is 124, and the average YPLL is 24.8.

The functional relationship between age and YPLL is shown in **FIGURE 1.5**, with each value falling directly on the line, which is a characteristic of a functional relationship.

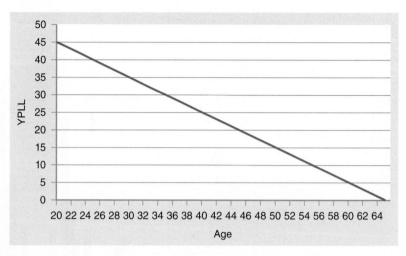

FIGURE 1.5 Functional relationship between variables Age and YPLL

1. $X \rightarrow Y \rightarrow Z$ Y is a mediator for X and Z
2. $X \leftarrow Y \leftarrow Z$ Y is a mediator for Z and X
3. $X \rightarrow Y \leftarrow Z$ Both X and Z cause Y; the path between X and Z is blocked
4. $X \leftarrow Y \rightarrow Z$ Y is a cause of X and of Z
5. $X \rightarrow Z$ Y is a confounder of the association between X and Z
   $\nwarrow \nearrow$
   Y

FIGURE 1.6 Path diagram

On the other hand, a **statistical relationship** is not a perfect one, in that all observations do not generally fall on the curve of relationship. Instead, there is a scattering of points around the line conveying the statistical relationship. For example, suppose you are interested in measuring the effect of age on muscle mass. For a given sample, you find that as age goes up, muscle mass goes down in a linear fashion. However, not all observations fall on the line, indicating that only some, not all, of the variation in muscle mass is accounted for by age. In epidemiology, the concept of an association between variables, such as an exposure and health outcome, is a familiar one. This relationship is typically not a perfect one.

Evidence from experience, observation, or experiment provides information about potential exposures and health outcome variables, as well as variables that may confound, mediate, or moderate relationships between exposure and outcome variables. The study investigator decides how a variable will be treated in a model: as an exposure, outcome, confounder, mediator, or moderator. A **confounder** yields a hidden effect on the outcome variable, a **mediator** is intermediate in the causal connection between the exposure and outcome variables, and a **moderator** is a variable that affects the strength of the relationship between an exposure and outcome variable. Causal diagrams are sometimes used to show the relationship between variables (such as X, Y, and Z) where a confounder, mediator, or moderator is involved (**FIGURE 1.6**).

▸ Statistical Modeling

Measures of statistical strength of association among variables of interest can be described and analyzed mathematically, depending on the type of data involved. Statistical models used to measure the strength of the association between exposure and outcome variables can adjust for potential confounding variables by including these variables in the model. For example, in a recent study finding support for an association between particulate air pollution, reasoning, and memory decline, researchers adjusted for time, age, sex, ethnicity, socioeconomic position, physical activity level, and alcohol use in a statistical model.[22] The statistical model also included an interaction term to determine whether the association between particulate air pollution and reasoning and memory decline was modified by age. The effect of mediating variables on exposure-outcome variables can also be quantitatively assessed using statistical models.

In general, **statistical modeling** in epidemiology involves the activity of translating a real public health problem into mathematics for subsequent analysis. Statistical models describe patterns of association and interactions in data. They allow us to evaluate variables that predict or explain the outcome variable of interest and whether variables modify this relationship. Mediating variables may be assessed in these models. In the context of an infectious disease, a statistical model can help us understand and possibly control the spread of the disease.

Summary

1. Epidemiology involves the study of the distribution and determinants of disease, events, behaviors, and existing conditions. The distribution of a health-related state or event involves its frequency and pattern. Identifying determinants assumes that health-related states or events do not occur at random and that causal and preventive factors can be identified through study.

2. Descriptive methods are used in epidemiology to monitor health states and exposures, determining whether a health problem exists, identifying those at greatest risk, and revealing when and where the health problem is most pronounced.

3. Analytic methods are used in epidemiology to assess whether a given exposure is associated with a disease or other health-related outcome. Descriptive and analytic epidemiologic information contributes to preventing and controlling diseases and other health problems.

4. Mathematical operations are used in epidemiology to (1) track the progress of infectious disease, the virulence of disease, and the persistence of pathogens in their hosts; (2) monitor the success rates of interventions; (3) test hypotheses; (4) quantify relationships among variables; (5) determine the appropriate sample size; and (6) communicate health findings.

5. Numbers are arithmetic values that are used in counting, making calculations, identifying subjects, and showing a position in a series.

6. An equation is a statement wherein the values of two mathematical expressions are equal. A formula is a special type of equation that shows the relationship between different variables.

7. GIS is a computer technique that combines spatial information with one or more layers of attribute information (characteristics of the objects under investigation).

8. An epidemic curve is a graph of the frequency of disease by time, showing the course of the health problem. The graph shows where the frequency distribution has its peak (central location), the spread of the data around the peak (spread), and whether the distribution of data is symmetric on both sides of the peak.

9. A functional relationship associates an input variable with an output variable. Change in the output variable is completely explained by change in the input variable. In contrast, a statistical relationship is not a perfect one.

10. The study investigator decides, based on experience, how a variable will be treated in a model: as an exposure, outcome, confounder, mediator, or moderator. A confounder produces a hidden effect on the outcome variable, a mediator is intermediate in the causal process between the exposure and outcome variables, and a moderator is a variable that affects the strength of the relationship between the exposure and outcome variables.

11. Modeling in epidemiology involves the activity of translating a real public health problem into mathematics for subsequent analysis. The mathematics can describe patterns of association and interactions in the data.

Computer Application

Microsoft Excel, Epi Info™ 7, and selected online interactive programs will be used for exercises in this book. Microsoft Excel was developed by Microsoft for Windows, Mac OS, Android, and iOS. It features the ability to store, organize, and manipulate data (i.e., make calculations, graphs, and more). It is used to create spreadsheets, which are special documents that allow us to store and organize data in rows (horizontal sets of boxes labeled as 1, 2, 3, and so on) and columns (vertical sets of boxes labeled as A, B, C, and so on). This data can then be read and manipulated. The intersection of each row and column is a cell wherein we enter numbers, text, or formulas.

An Excel document is a workbook. A workbook consists of one or more worksheets. Worksheets are the grid where we store and calculate data. Simple and complex formulas can be calculated in Excel. Excel also offers a variety of charts (e.g., line graph, bar chart, scatter plot) to assess data.

1. Epi Info™ consists of free data management, analysis, and visualization tools for public health. It is a series of programs for Microsoft Windows that are useful for epidemiologists and other public health professionals in carrying out outbreak investigations, managing databases, performing statistical analyses, mapping and visualizing data, and developing summary reports.

    Epi Info 7, the latest version, is free of charge and can be downloaded from the CDC website by searching for "Epi Info" on the CDC homepage. Click the Download option and then download the program to your desktop. Select "Open" (or "Run") when prompted.

    Epi Info 7 provides the following tools: Form Designer, which is used to create a questionnaire or form to collect and view data; Enter, which is used to show existing records or to enter data; Classic Analysis, which is used to perform statistical analyses and create tables, graphs, and charts; Map, which is used to create maps; Options, which is used for constructing custom configurations; and StatCalc, which is used for summarizing, describing, and evaluating data.

    An instructional video on Epi Info 7 can be found on the CDC's YouTube channel.

2. In this chapter, we calculated a measure of risk, called the "attack rate." We also calculated a person-time rate and a prevalence proportion. Open the Excel workbook Application 1.1.xlsx. Move your cursor to cell C7 and double-click the mouse. You will then see the formula typed into the

cell to obtain the attack rate. Similarly, go to other cells, such as K4, K5, K6, K8, K9, K11, and N8, and double-click each of these cells to see the formulas to type in order to obtain the values shown in the spreadsheet.

3. For the 40 cases in the first problem, suppose we are interested in graphing the epidemic curve. Open the Excel workbook Application 1.2.xlsx. To create a graph of this data, move your cursor to cell C2, click the mouse, and drag the cursor down through C12. Then go to the Insert tab, go to the Charts icon (horizontal column chart), place the mouse over the first 2-D column graph, and click the mouse. This will create a histogram. In the graph, click the horizontal axis, and under the Design tab, click Select Data. Then choose Edit. Put the mouse at cell B2, click, and drag the cursor through B12. Then select OK. You will be prompted to select OK again. You have now successfully relabeled the horizontal axis. Now click the chart and go to the Add Chart Element tab on the upper-left side of the screen. Click and go to Axis Titles. Choose Primary Vertical, highlight the Axis Title, and type "Number"; then choose Primary Horizontal, highlight the Axis Title, and type "Hour"; then replace "Chart Title" with "Epidemic curve showing cases by time."

4. Open the Excel workbook Application 1.3.xlsx. Here you can see the data table used to compute the total YPLL and the average YPLL. See if you can recreate the empty cells for the table. To recreate Figure 1.5, take the cursor to cell H3 (notice how the value in the cell was calculated), click the mouse, and drag the cursor down through H48. Then go to the Insert tab, go to the Charts icon (line chart), and put the mouse over the first 2-D line graph. In the graph, select the horizontal axis and go to the Select Data tab. Then choose Edit. Put the mouse at cell G3, click the mouse, and drag the cursor through G48. Then select OK. You will be prompted to select OK again. You have now successfully relabeled the horizontal axis. Now click the chart and go to the Add Chart Element tab on the toolbar. Click and go to Axis Titles. Select titles for the horizontal axis and the vertical axis. Also, add a title.

5. Go to the following website and create your own map. https://datamapper .geo.census.gov/map.html

6. Once you have downloaded Epi Info 7, click on the icon to start. Then select Create Maps. The CDC has a tutorial on maps that you can find in the Epi Info user guide. Create your own map.

References

1. Doll, R. (1998). Epidemiological evidence of the effects of behavior and the environment on the risk of human cancer. *Recent Results in Cancer Research. 154,* 3–21.
2. Lipsey, S. (1993). Mathematical education in the life of Florence Nightingale. *Biographies of Women Mathematicians.* Retrieved from https://www.agnesscott.edu/lriddle/women/night _educ.htm.
3. Daniel, T. M. (2005). Wade Hampton Frost, pioneer epidemiologist 1880–1938: Up to the mountain. American Journal of Epidemiology, *162(3),* 290–291.
4. Doll, R., & Hill, A. B. (1956). Lung cancer and other causes of death in relation to smoking: a second report on the mortality of British doctors. *British Medical Journal, 2* (5001): 1071–1081.
5. Miettinen, O. S. (1969). Individual matching with multiple controls in the case of all-or-none responses. *Biometrics, 22,* 339–355.
6. Miettinen, O. S. (1975). *Principles of epidemiologic research* (Unpublished manuscript). Harvard University, Cambridge, MA.
7. Miettinen, O. S. (1976). Estimability and estimation in case-referent studies. *American Journal of Epidemiology, 103(2),* 226–235.
8. Miettinen, O. S., & Wang, J. D. (1981). An alternative to the proportionate mortality ratio. *American Journal of Epidemiology, 114,* 144–148.

9. Greenhouse, S. W., Greenhouse, J. B., & Cornfield, J. (2005). In *Encyclopedia of biostatistics*. New York: John Wiley & Sons.

10. Scott, W. (1955). Reliability of content analysis: The case of nominal scale coding. *Public Opinion Quarterly*, *19(3)*, 321–325.

11. Fleiss, J. L. (1971). Measuring nominal scale agreement among many raters. *Psychology Bulletin*, *76(5)*, 378–382.

12. Day, N. E., & Gail, M. H. (2007). Norman Breslow, an architect of modern biostatistics. *Lifetime Data Anal*; doi:10.1007/s10985-007-9052-2. Retrieved from https://pdfs .semanticscholar.org/ae65/b6f01a5cf902894364e2da58025285d74df2.pdf

13. Cochran, W. G., & Cox, G. M. (1992). *Experimental designs* (2nd ed.). New York: John Wiley & Sons.

14. Cochran, W. G. (1977). *Sampling techniques* (3rd ed.). New York: John Wiley & Sons.

15. Snedecor, G. W., & Cochran, W. G. (1956). *Statistical methods, applied to experiments in agriculture and biology* (5th ed.). Ames, IA: Iowa State College Press.

16. Moses, L. E., & Mosteller, F., (Eds.). (1983). *Planning and analysis of observational studies*. New York: John Wiley & Sons.

17. Kleinbaum, D. G., Kupper, L. L., & Morgenstern, H. (1982). *Epidemiologic research: principles and quantitative methods*. New York: John Wiley & Sons.

18. Merrill, R. M. (2017). *Introduction to epidemiology* (7th ed.). Burlington, MA: Jones & Bartlett Learning.

19. Hippocrates. Airs, waters, places. In Buck, C., Llopis, A., Najera, E., & Terris, M., (Eds.). (1988). *The challenge of epidemiology: Issues and selected readings*. Washington, DC: World Health Organization, 18–19.

20. Snow, J. (1855). *On the mode of communication of cholera* (2nd ed.). London: John Churchill.

21. Ray, N., & Ebener, S., (2008). AccessMod 3.0: Computing geographic coverage and accessibility to health care services using anisotropic movement of patients. *International Journal of Health Geographics, 7*, 63.

22. Tonne, C., Elbas, A., Beevers, S., & Singh-Manoux, A. (2014). Traffic-related air pollution in relation to cognitive function in older adults. *Epidemiology, 25(5)*, 674–681.

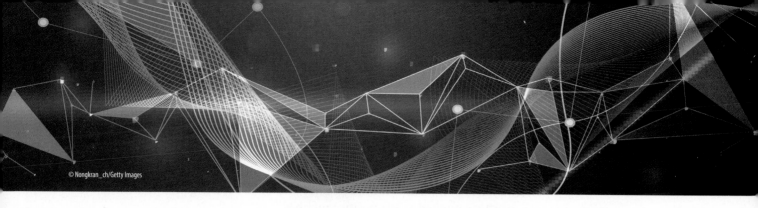

CHAPTER 2

Arithmetic and Algebra in Epidemiology

The most elementary branch of mathematics is **arithmetic**, which is the study of numbers, particularly operations between numbers. Basic operations of arithmetic include addition, subtraction, multiplication, and division. More advanced operations of arithmetic include percentages, square roots, exponentiation, and logarithmic functions. Whereas arithmetic involves the computation of specific numbers, **algebra** uses letters and other symbols to represent numbers that are either unknown or that can assume many values, according to the rules of arithmetic. Algebra represents what is true in many situations for all numbers. An example of an arithmetic expression is $3 + 5$. An example of an algebraic expression is $3 + x$.

The purpose of this chapter is to present the real number system, the number line, arithmetic and algebra properties, the order of operations, fractions, exponents and roots, the laws of exponents, and logarithms.

▶ Real Number System

In the previous chapter, we introduced some important uses of numbers in epidemiology. The numbers we use in epidemiology, as well as in everyday life, are referred to as "real numbers". **Real numbers** are values that represent quantities on a number line. The most familiar ones are **integers** (also called "whole numbers"), which are the numbers 0, 1, −1, 2, −2, …, and so on. The real number system also includes rational numbers. **Rational numbers** consist of all fractions of the ratio or quotient of two integers (a/b), where a and b are integers and $b \neq 0$. Some real numbers are not rational numbers; an **irrational number** is a number that cannot be expressed as the ratio of two integers. Some common irrational numbers are $\pi = 3.14159\ldots = ?/?$ (no ratio), $e = 2.71828\ldots = ?/?$ (no ratio), and many square roots, cube roots, and so on (e.g., $\sqrt{2} = ?/?$) (no ratio).

▶ The Number Line

On a **number line**, every real number has a unique point (**FIGURE 2.1**). In converse, every point on the number line contains a unique real number label. For any real number, those to the right of 0 on the number line are positive numbers (all numbers a with $a > 0$), and all numbers to the left of 0 on the number line are negative numbers (all numbers b with $b < 0$). Nonnegative numbers are all numbers a with $a \geq 0$. If c is a positive number, $-c$ is a negative number; if c is a negative number, $-c$ is a positive number.

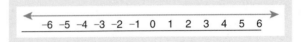

FIGURE 2.1 Number line

Order Relation and the Operations of Arithmetic

1. If $a \leq b$, then $a + c \leq b + c$
2. If $a \leq b$ and $c > 0$, then $ac \leq bc$
3. If $a \leq b$ and $c < 0$, then $ac \geq bc$
4. If $a \leq b$, then $\dfrac{1}{a} \geq \dfrac{1}{b}$

▶ Properties (or Laws) of Arithmetic and Algebraic Operations

The operations of addition, subtraction, multiplication, division, and exponentiation work the same way in arithmetic and algebra; the only difference is that arithmetic operations are performed on numbers, and algebraic operations are performed on variables. It is important to understand the meaning of the properties (or laws) of arithmetic and algebraic operations in order to apply these in different situations. These math properties will be presented here.

Negatives of Real Numbers

1. $c + (-c) = 0$
2. $-(-c) = c$
3. $(-1) \times c = -c$
4. $b + (-c) = b - c$
5. $-(b + c) = -b - c$
6. $b - (-c) = b + c$

Signs If b and c Are Any Real Number

1. $(-b)(-c) = bc$
2. $-b(c) = b(-c) = -bc$
3. $\dfrac{-b}{-c} = \dfrac{b}{c} (c \neq 0)$
4. $\dfrac{-b}{c} = \dfrac{b}{-c} = -\dfrac{b}{c} (c \neq 0)$

Commutative Laws for Any Real Number
1. $b + c = c + b$
2. $bc = cb$

Associative Laws for Any Real Number
1. $b + (c + d) = (b + c) + d$
2. $b(cd) = bc(d)$

Distributive Laws for Any Real Number
1. $b(c + d) = bc + bd, (c + d)b = cb + db$
2. $b(c - d)bc - bd, (c - d)b = cb - db$

Zero Products for Any Real Number
1. $b \times 0 = 0 = 0 \times b$
2. If $cd = 0, c = 0$ or $d = 0$ (or both)
3. If $c \neq 0$ and $d \neq 0$, then $cd \neq 0$

▶ Basic Properties of Absolute Values

There are situations in epidemiologic studies in which the absolute value is involved, such as when considering tests of significance, like the t statistic ($|t| > t$ (critical value)), or the chi-square statistic, where some forms of the statistic include a measure of absolute value. The basic properties of absolute values are presented.

$$|c| \geq 0 \text{ and } |c| > 0 \text{ when } c \neq 0$$

$$|c| = |-c|$$

$$|c|^2 = c^2 = |c^2|$$

$$\sqrt{c^2} = |c|$$

$$|cd| = |c||d| \text{ and if } d \neq 0, \left|\frac{c}{d}\right| = \frac{|c|}{|d|}$$

$|c|$ is the distance between c and 0 on the number line.

If k is a positive number, then the only numbers with absolute value k are k and $-k$.

The distance between the numbers c and d on the number line is the number $|c - d|$.

Absolute value is the distance from zero on a number line. This value is always positive.

$$|5| = 5$$

$$|-3| = 3$$

$$|3^2 - 20| = 11$$

▶ Fractions

Addition and Subtraction

$$\frac{a}{b} + \frac{c}{b} = \frac{a+c}{b} \qquad\qquad \frac{a}{b} - \frac{c}{b} = \frac{a-c}{b} \quad b \neq 0$$

$$\frac{a}{b} + \frac{c}{d} = \frac{ad}{bd} + \frac{bc}{bd} \qquad\qquad \frac{a}{b} - \frac{c}{d} = \frac{ad}{bd} - \frac{bc}{bd}$$

$$= \frac{ad+bc}{bd} \quad b \neq 0, d \neq 0 \qquad\qquad = \frac{ad-bc}{bd} \quad b \neq 0, d \neq 0$$

Multiplication of Fractions

$$\frac{a}{b} \times \frac{c}{d} = \frac{ac}{bd} \quad b \neq 0, d \neq 0$$

Division of Fractions

$$\frac{a}{c/d} = \frac{a}{1} \times \frac{d}{c} = \frac{ad}{c} \quad c \neq 0, d \neq 0 \qquad\qquad \frac{a/b}{c} = \frac{a}{b} \times \frac{1}{c} = \frac{a}{bc} \quad b \neq 0, c \neq 0$$

$$\frac{a/b}{c/d} = \frac{a}{b} \times \frac{d}{c} = \frac{ad}{bc} \quad b \neq 0, c \neq 0, d \neq 0$$

▶ Order of Operations

Arithmetic is performed according to a collection of rules that define an order of operation. The order of operation must be followed to avoid making arithmetic mistakes. First, do all computations inside the parentheses before doing computations outside the parentheses. Second, when parentheses are within parentheses, work from the inside out. Third, multiplication and division are performed first, followed by addition and subtraction.

P	E	M	D	A	S
Please	Excuse	My	Dear	Aunt	Sally
Parentheses	Exponents	Multiplication Division Work from left to right $\rightarrow$		Addition Subtraction Work from left to right $\rightarrow$	
( ) [ ] { }	$\sqrt{a} = a^{1/2}, a^2, e^n$	$\times$	$\div$	$+$	$-$

▶ Exponents and Roots

An **exponent** is a quantity that reflects the power to which a number or expression is raised, such as 2 in $4^2 = 16$; it provides a notational shorthand approach for certain products.

If c is a real number and n is a positive integer, c^n is the product of c n times (n factors).

If c is a real number that does not equal zero, then $c^0 = 1$.

For a given nonzero real number c and a positive integer n, $c^{-n} = 1/c^n$.

For nonzero real numbers c and d and integers m and n,

I. $c^m c^n = c^{m+n}$

II. $\dfrac{c^m}{c^n} = c^{m-n}$

III. $(c^m)^n = c^{mn}$

IV. $(cd)^n = c^n d^n$

V. $\left(\dfrac{c}{d}\right)^n = \dfrac{c^n}{d^n}$

VI. $\dfrac{1}{c^{-n}} = c^n$

▶ Laws of Exponents

For nonnegative real numbers c and d and positive integers m and n,

I. $c^{1/n} = \sqrt[n]{c}$

II. $c^{n/m} = \left(\sqrt[m]{c}\right)^n = \sqrt[m]{c^n}$

III. $\left(\sqrt[n]{d}\right)^n = \left(\sqrt[n]{d^n}\right) = d^{n/n} = d$

IV. $\sqrt[m]{\sqrt[n]{d}} = \sqrt[mn]{d}$

V. $\sqrt[n]{cd} = \sqrt[n]{c}\sqrt[n]{d}$

VI. $\sqrt[n]{\dfrac{c}{d}} = \dfrac{\sqrt[n]{c}}{\sqrt[n]{d}} \ (d \neq 0)$

▶ Exponential Functions

A function involves a relationship in which each input has a single output, such as $y = f(x) = x^2$, where the base x is variable and the fixed number 2 is the power. On the other hand, with exponentials the base is a fixed number and the power is variable, such as $y = g(x) = 2^x$. This is shown in **FIGURE 2.2**.

x	$y = 2^x$
−3	0.125
−2	0.25
−1	0.5

(continues)

x	$y = 2^x$
0	1
1	2
2	4
3	8

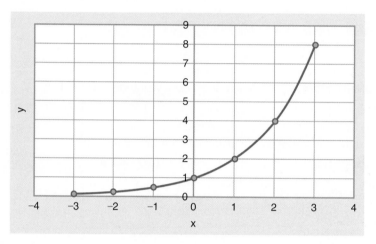

FIGURE 2.2 Graph showing the exponential function

In epidemiology, populations, exposures, and health-related states or events may increase or decrease exponentially over time. The exponential growth and decay formula is

$$y = f(x) = ab^x$$

where $a \neq 0$, the base $b \neq 1$, and x is any real number. In this function, a is the starting value (e.g., the initial population or dosage level), and b is the growth or decay factor. If $b > 1$, the function represents exponential growth. If $0 < b < 1$, the function represents exponential decline. If r represents the rate of increase or its decrease expressed as a decimal,

$b = 1 - r$; decay $= (1 - r)^2$
$b = 1 + r$; growth $= (1 + r)^2$
A rate of decrease of 10% is a decay factor of $b = 1 - 0.10 = 0.90$.
A rate of increase of 20% is a growth factor of $b = 1 + 0.20 = 1.20$.
The variable x indicates how many times the growth or decay factor is multiplied.

The rate of increase or decrease is calculated as Present/Past $- 1$.

The formulas just described assume that growth and decay happen in discrete steps; that is, growth is instantaneous at the end of each time interval. Consider the growth formula at the end of one year, growth $= 1 + r$. If r is 100%, then growth $= 1 + 1 = 2$. However, if the formula used two periods in our growth equation, growth $= \left(1 + 1/2\right)^2 = 2.25$, or 100 periods in our growth equation, growth $= \left(1 + 1/100\right)^{100} = 2.7048$, or 1,000,000 periods in our growth equation, growth $= \left(1 + 1/1,000,000\right)^{1,000,000} = 2.71828$. In general, as n gets larger and larger, the growth formula approaches 2.71828..., which is an important irrational number in mathematics called e.

If the rate of inrease $r = 50\%$ and we choose $n = 50$, then growth $= (+0.50/50)^{50} = (1 + 0.01)^{50} = 1.6446$. But notice that $(1 + 0.01)^{50} = (1 + 0.01)^{100/2} = \left[(1 + 0.01)^{100}\right]^{1/2} = 2.7048^{1/2} = 1.6446$. If we increase the periods in our growth formula to a very large number, then growth $= e^{\text{rate}}$.

Suppose we have a 200% rate of increase for one year, then growth $= e^2$. For two years, growth $= \left(e^2\right)^2 = e^4$. As a general rule, growth $= \left(e^{\text{rate}}\right)^{\text{time}} = e^{rt}$. Hence, an alternative population growth model to that described earlier is

$$y = f(x) = ae^{rt}$$

▶ Logarithms

Several analytic procedures in epidemiology use exponential and logarithmic functions. Logarithms are closely related to exponential functions. Consider that $y = a^x$ is equivalent to $\log_a y = x$, where $\log_a y$ is the base a logarithm of y; the number of times we multiply a to get y is equal to x. For example, how many 2s do we multiply to get 16? The answer is $2 \times 2 \times 2 \times 2 = 16$, so the logarithm is 4, written as $\log_2 16 = 4$. In other words, log base 2 of 16 is 4.

Different base values can be used, but the most common are 10 and e (i.e., 2.71828...). Logarithms of base 10 are called **common logarithms**. Logarithms of base e are called **natural logarithms**. Base 10 is used more frequently in the fields of engineering and chemistry. Base e is used in calculus because it is easily integrated and differentiated. Mathematical answers come out naturally (hence the term "natural log," abbreviated as ln), as opposed to requiring additional coefficients when base 10 is used.

Two important properties of logarithms are

$a^{\log_a y} = y$ for every positive real number y

$\log_a(a^x) = x$ for every real number x

The following are restatements of the laws of exponents, but in terms of logarithms:

$$\log_a(xy) = \log_a x + \log_a y \text{ for all positive real numbers } x, y.$$

$$\log_a\left(\frac{x}{y}\right) = \log_a x - \log_a y \text{ for all positive real numbers } x, y.$$

$$\log_a(x^k) = k(\log_a x) \text{ for all real numbers } k \text{ and } x \text{ with } x > 0.$$

Several measures in epidemiology use logarithms. Some of these are listed here.

1. The Estimated Annual Percent Change (EAPC) in rates is calculated by fitting a regression line to the natural logarithm of the rates, where $\ln(\text{rate}) = a + b \times \text{Year}$. The EAPC $= 100(e^b - 1)$.
2. In logistic regression, the outcome variable is transformed using the natural log, $\ln\left(p/1 - p\right)$. If the outcome variable in epidemiology takes on the values 1 or 0, with probability p and $1 - p$, respectively, then the outcome variable does not satisfy certain assumptions used in regression analysis.

3. Poisson regression analysis is appropriate for studying rare diseases in large populations. In Poisson regression, the outcome variable is transformed using the natural log, ln(rate).

4. Confidence intervals for common epidemiologic measures of association, such as odds ratio, risk ratio, rate ratio, and prevalence ratio.

5. Change in the natural log is approximately equal to the percent change. Hence, to get a sense as to the percent change in rates over time, we can use a semi-log graph, which is defined by a logarithmic scale on the vertical axis and a linear scale on the horizontal axis. A straight line reflects a constant rate of change. For example, the annual percent change in melanoma in the United States for males and females is shown in **FIGURE 2.3**. The percent change is increasing but at a decreasing rate of change. Note that the log scale with base e is 2.7 ($=2.7^1$), 7.29 ($=2.7^2$), 19.683 ($=2.7^3$), and 53.1441 ($=2.7^4$).

6. A model with a logarithmic transformation of years 1–36 fits the decreasing trend in lead concentrations in the United States from 1980–2015 (**FIGURE 2.4**).

7. A model with an exponential transformation of age groups (1–10) fits the increasing death rates of diabetes mellitus with older age (**FIGURE 2.5**).

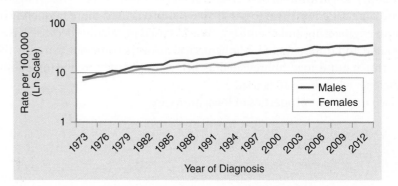

FIGURE 2.3 Melanoma in whites, United States

Data from: Surveillance, Epidemiology, and End Results (SEER) Program (www.seer.cancer.gov) SEER*Stat Database: Mortality—All COD, Aggregated with State, Total U.S. (1969–2013) <Katrina/Rita Population Adjustment>, National Cancer Institute, DCCPS, Surveillance Research Program, Surveillance Systems Branch, released April 2016.

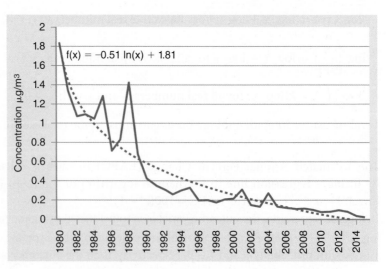

FIGURE 2.4 Lead air quality, 1980–2015 (annual maximum three-month average), United States

Data from: https://www.epa.gov/air-trends/lead-trends

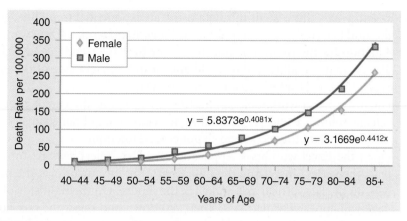

FIGURE 2.5 Death rates for diabetes mellitus in the United States, 2011–2013

Data from: Surveillance, Epidemiology, and End Results (SEER) Program (www.seer.cancer.gov) SEER*Stat Database: Mortality—All COD, Aggregated with State, Total U.S. (1969–2013) <Katrina/Rita Population Adjustment>, National Cancer Institute, DCCPS, Surveillance Research Program, Surveillance Systems Branch, released April 2016. Underlying mortality data provided by NCHS (www.cdc.gov/nchs).

Summary

1. Arithmetic involves the computation of specific numbers. Algebra uses letters or other symbols to represent numbers that are either unknown or that can assume many values according to the rules of arithmetic. Algebra represents what is true in many situations for all numbers.
2. Real numbers represent quantities on a number line, the most familiar being integers, which are whole numbers (0, −1, 1, −2, 2, …).
3. Every real number has a unique point on a number line.
4. Several arithmetic properties (or laws) were presented, including cumulative laws, associative laws, and distributive laws for any real number, along with a collection of rules that define an order of operation. These laws and the order of operation work the same way between arithmetic and algebra, and they must be followed to avoid making computational mistakes.
5. The order of operation is parentheses, exponents, multiplication, division, addition, and subtraction.
6. With exponentials, the base is a fixed number and the power is variable. For example, the exponential growth model is $y = f(x) = ae^{rt}$, where r is the rate of growth and t is time.
7. A logarithm is a value that represents the power that a fixed number (base) is raised to produce a number; the number of times we multiply a to get y is equal to x, written as $\log_a y = x$, and equivalent to the exponential function $y = a^x$. Two common logarithms involve base 10 (called "common logarithms") and base e (called "natural logarithms").

Computer Application

1. Open the Excel workbook Application 2.1.xlsx. Put the cursor over each cell to see how we obtained the values. The values in this spreadsheet match the problems in this chapter, up through the section on Exponential Functions.
2. Open the Excel workbook Application 2.2.xlsx. Highlight the data, then go to Insert, and then Charts. Select Scatter and the first graph. Select the graph and then choose Design. Go to the Add Chart Element and add the

x- and *y*-axis titles. To fit this data using an exponential trend line, go to the Add Chart Element, Trendline, and then Exponential. If you want the equation for the trend line, put the cursor over the trend line and click. The Format Trendline options will appear on the right side of the page. Select the box Display Equation on the chart.

3.   Open the Excel workbook Application 2.3.xlsx. Put the cursor over the cells in column F and H3, J3, and L3 to see how we obtained answers to the problems in the section on Exponential Functions.

4.   Open the Excel workbook Application 2.4.xlsx. Select cells B2 through D43, then select Insert and the Line Chart. Put the cursor over the numbers on the left vertical axis and click the mouse. On the right side of the page will appear Format Axis. There, go down and select the box Logarithmic Scale and type "e" in the box. This will give you the plot based on the natural logarithm. Add a chart title and a left axis title.

Practice Problems

2.1

Express the following statements as symbols.

−5 is greater than −10 _____

a is nonnegative _____

b lies strictly between −2 and −1 _____

c is less than 5 and *d* is at least 5 _____

2.2

For each of the following statements, insert ≤, ≥, <, or > in the blank to make the statement true.

If $a \leq b < 0$, $\dfrac{1}{a}$ _____ $\dfrac{1}{b}$

If $0 \leq a < b$, a^2 _____ b^2

If $a \leq 0 \leq b$, a^3 _____ b^3

2.3

Find the negatives of each of the following numbers (express as a number or symbol).

$-\pi$ _____

$[6 + (-8)]$ _____

$[80 - (90 - 5)]$ _____

$-2\pi(10 - \pi)$ _____

2.4

Express each of the following as a single number.

$(-20)(-5)$ _____

$(-30 + 40)(-5)$ _____

$\dfrac{-14}{-7}$ _____

$\dfrac{0}{-14}$ _____

2.5

Provide an example showing there is no cumulative law for subtraction.

_____

2.6

Provide an example showing there is no cumulative law for division.

_____

2.7

Provide an example showing there is no associative law for subtraction.

_____

2.8

Provide an example showing there is no associative law for division.

_____

2.9

Solve $(x - 3)(x - 2) = 0$.

_____

2.10

What is the effect size for the correlation coefficient −0.25? _____

2.11

What is the distance from −2 to 2? _____

2.12

In the United States, approximately 1 out of 20 deaths is attributed to accidents and 1 out of 4 deaths is attributed to heart disease. How many deaths are attributed to accidents and heart disease?

_____

2.13

In the United States, there is one birth every 8 seconds, one death every 12 seconds, and one international migrant (net) every 33 seconds. How many seconds does it take for a net gain of one person?

_____

2.14

Approximately 227 per 1,000 adults in the United States have doctor-diagnosed arthritis. For every 19 men with arthritis, there are 26 women with the disease. What is the number of men with arthritis per 1,000 people?

_____

What is the number of women with arthritis per 1,000 people?

_____

2.15

In the United States, an estimated 1 in 8 women will develop breast cancer over her lifetime and 1 in 6 men will develop prostate cancer. The risk of prostate cancer in men compared with the risk of breast cancer in women is _____ times greater or _____ percent higher.

2.16

Compute the following and express as a single number.

$$\left(\frac{48}{2}\right) - 4^2 + 2 \times 2z$$

$$\frac{(-2)\left(\dfrac{2+2}{3-5}\right) + 6^2 - 1}{-2 + 10\left(\dfrac{8-10}{12-16}\right)}$$

2.17

Regarding the laws of exponents, show that these six equations hold for $c = 2$, $d = 5$, $m = 3$, and $n = 4$.

I. $c^m c^n = c^{m+n}$

II. $\dfrac{c^m}{c^n} = c^{m-n}$

III. $(c^m)^n = c^{mn}$

IV. $(cd)^n = c^n d^n$

V. $\left(\dfrac{c}{d}\right)^n = \dfrac{c^n}{d^n}$

VI. $\dfrac{1}{c^{-n}} = c^n$

I.   _____

II.   _____

III.   _____

IV.   _____

V.   _____

VI.   _____

2.18

Show that these six laws of exponents hold for $c = 2$, $d = 5$, $m = 3$, and $n = 4$.

I. $c^{1/n} = \sqrt[n]{c}$

II. $c^{n/m} = \left(\sqrt[m]{c}\right)^n = \sqrt[m]{c^n}$

III. $\left(\sqrt[n]{d}\right)^n = \left(\sqrt[n]{d^n}\right) = d^{n/n} = d$

IV. $\sqrt[m]{\sqrt[n]{d}} = \sqrt[mn]{d}$

V. $\sqrt[n]{cd} = \sqrt[n]{c}\sqrt[n]{d}$

VI. $\sqrt[n]{\dfrac{c}{d}} = \dfrac{\sqrt[n]{c}}{\sqrt[n]{d}} \ (d \neq 0)$

I.   _____

II.   _____

III.   _____

IV.   _____

V.   _____

VI.   _____

2.19

What is the rate of increase for the following top 10 states in percent growth from 2015 to 2016? Round your answer to four places after the decimal.

Rank	Name	2015	2016	r
1	Utah	2,990,632	3,051,217	_____
2	Nevada	2,883,758	2,940,058	_____
3	Idaho	1,652,828	1,683,140	_____
4	Florida	20,244,914	20,612,439	_____
5	Washington	7,160,290	7,288,000	_____
6	Oregon	4,024,634	4,093,465	_____
7	Colorado	5,448,819	5,540,545	_____
8	Arizona	6,817,565	6,931,071	_____
9	District of Columbia	670,377	681,170	_____
10	Texas	27,429,639	27,862,596	_____

Data source: https://www.census.gov/newsroom/press-releases/2016/cb16-214.html

2.20

Refer to the table in Problem 2.19. Assuming the rate of increase in the Utah population stays constant through 2050, what is the estimated population in that year? _____

2.21

Refer to the table in Problem 2.19. Assuming the rate of increase in the Utah population stays constant through 2050, what is the estimated population in that year, based on this alternative population growth model? _____

2.22

A patient is given a 500 mg dose of medicine that degrades by 30% per hour. What is the drug concentration in the patient after 24 hours? Round your answer to three places after the decimal.

_____ mg

2.23

Using the correct options from below, complete the following table.

Logarithmic Form	
	$y = a^x$
$\log_3 9 = 2$	
	$27 = 3^3$
$\log_4 \dfrac{1}{16} = -2$	

$\log_y a = x$

$9 = 2^3$

$9 = 3^2$

$\log_a y = x$

$\dfrac{1}{16} = 4^{-2}$

$\log_3 27 = 3$

$4^{-16/2}$

$\log_3 3 = 27$

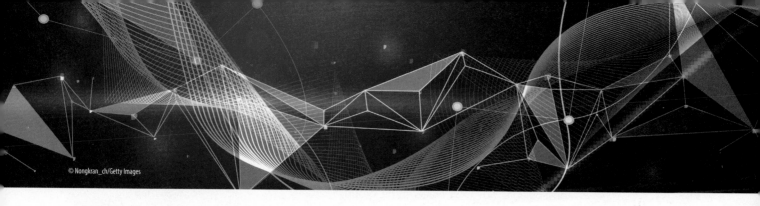

CHAPTER 3

Descriptive Statistical Measures in Epidemiology

At the beginning of this book we defined "statistics" as the science of data, a branch of mathematics that involves collecting, classifying, summarizing, organizing, analyzing, and interpreting data. Statistics can be divided into four general areas: descriptive, probability, inferential, and statistical techniques. The purpose of this chapter is to provide an overview of descriptive statistics and its use in epidemiology.

▶ Scales of Measurement

Part of the role of epidemiology is to study the distribution of health-related states or events in the population. The scale of measurement represents the precision wherein an attribute is measured. The scale in which an attribute is measured has implications for the way the information is summarized and described. There are three scales of measurement: nominal, ordinal, and numerical. These scales of measurement are presented in **TABLE 3.1**, along with common statistics and graphs used to summarize and describe the data.

Numerical data may be discrete or continuous. Discrete data can take on only those values that you can count (e.g., the number of occupants in a household, the number of people visiting the emergency room on a given day, or the number of disease cases in a community). Continuous data can take on any value within a range (e.g., a dose of radiation; a person's age, weight, or height). We will discuss numerical data in more detail shortly.

▶ Descriptive Measures: Nominal and Ordinal Data

Nominal and ordinal data are commonly presented using frequency and relative frequency tables. A **frequency distribution** is a tabular summary of a set

TABLE 3.1 Scales of Measurement

Scale	Description	Example	Statistics	Graphs
Nominal	Qualitative observations or categorical observations; no inherent ordering	Exposed (yes, no) Disease (yes, no) Sex Race/ethnic group Marital status Education level Income category	Frequency Relative frequency	Contingency tables Bar chart Spot map Area map
Ordinal	Qualitative observations or categorical observations; inherent ordering	Preference rating Rank-order scale	Frequency Relative frequency	Bar chart
Numerical	Quantitative observations; discrete (finite) and continuous (infinite) values	Dose of ionizing radiation Number of fractures	Geometric mean Arithmetic mean Median Mode Range Variance Standard deviation Coefficient of variation	Bar chart Histogram or frequency polygon

of data that shows the frequency or number of data items that fall in each of several distinct classes. A frequency distribution is also known as a "frequency table." The **relative frequency** of a category is the frequency of that category divided by the total number of observations.

$$\text{Relative frequency} = \frac{\text{Frequency}}{n}$$

n is the total number of observations (i.e., the sample size).

A **ratio** is a part divided by another part. It is the number of observations with the characteristic of interest divided by the number without the characteristic of interest. A **proportion** is the number of observations with the characteristic of interest divided by the total number of observations. It is used to summarize counts. Combining the frequency of cases for a selected time interval with the corresponding population at risk of becoming a case produces a rate, which is a special type of proportion. A **rate** is a number of cases of a particular outcome divided by the size of the at-risk population in that time period, multiplied by a base (e.g., 100, 1,000, 10,000, or 100,000). The purpose of the rate base is to help us better understand, interpret, and communicate the result of our calculation. For example, instead of saying 0.35 of the people at a picnic were affected by salmonellosis, we can say 35 per 100 or 35% were affected. Another example involves female breast cancer where, in 2014, the rate of this disease in the United States was 0.00142. Rather than communicating this rate in its decimal form, we can multiply it by 100,000, and refer to the female breast cancer rate as 142 per 100,000. Cancer rates are usually reported per 100,000.

The algebraic expression for a ratio, proportion, or rate is

$$\frac{x}{y} \times 10^z$$

Here x refers to cases, y refers to the sample or population, and z is a whole number of 0 or greater.

We already presented formulas for measuring risk and prevalence. These measures fit the algebraic expression given here. Several descriptive measures are now presented for nominal scale data, shown in **TABLE 3.2** (morbidity), **TABLE 3.3** (mortality), and **TABLE 3.4** (natality).

The point prevalence proportion of arthritis is greater for adults who are obese (50% higher), have diabetes (70% higher), or have heart disease (90% higher), after adjustment for age (**FIGURE 3.1**).

▶ Descriptive Measures: Numerical Data

To summarize and describe numerical scale data, we use measures of central location (a single value that best represents a group who are described in a frequency distribution) and dispersion (variability, scatter, or spread). Before reviewing the common measures of central location and dispersion, some basic notation will be presented.

Capital letters are generally used to represent population data (a set or collection of items of interest in a study), and lowercase letters represent sample data (a subset of items that have been selected from the population). For example, X may represent the number of events of a nominal or ordinal variable in a population, such as the number of people exposed or the number of people who strongly agree. For discrete or continuous data, X_i is the ith observation in

TABLE 3.2 Measures of Morbidity

Measure	Numerator (*x*)	Denominator (*y*)	Expressed per Number at Risk (Rate Base)
Incidence rate	Number of new cases of a specified disease reported during a given time interval	Estimated population at mid-interval	Varies
Attack rate	Number of new cases of a specified disease reported during an epidemic period	Population at start of the epidemic period	Usually 100
Secondary attack rate	Number of new cases of a specified disease among contacts of known cases	Size of contact population at risk	Usually 100
Point prevalence proportion	Number of current cases, new and old, of a specified disease at a given point in time (a measure that reflects burden)	Estimated population at the same point in time	Usually 100

TABLE 3.3 Measures of Mortality

Measure	Numerator (x)	Denominator (y)	Expressed per Number at Risk (Rate Base)
Mortality rate	Total number of deaths reported during a given time interval	Estimated mid-interval population	1,000 or 100,000
Cause-specific death rate	Number of deaths assigned to a specific cause during a given time interval	Estimated mid-interval population	100,000
Proportional mortality ratio	Number of deaths assigned to a specific cause during a given time interval	Total number of deaths from all causes during the same time interval	100
Death-to-case ratio	Number of deaths assigned to a specific disease during a given time interval	Number of new cases of that disease reported during the same time interval	100
Neonatal mortality rate	Number of deaths under 28 days of age during a given time interval	Number of live births during the same time interval	1,000
Post-neonatal mortality rate	Number of deaths from 28 days upto, but not including, 1 year of age, during a given time interval	Number of live births during the same time interval	1,000
Infant mortality rate	Number of deaths under 1 year of age during a given time interval	Number of live births during the same time interval	1,000
Maternal mortality rate	Number of deaths assigned to pregnancy-related causes during a given time interval	Number of live births during the same time interval	100,000
Maternal mortality ratio	Number of deaths of women during or shortly after a pregnancy	100,000 live births	
Fetal death rate	Number of fetal deaths after at least 20 weeks of gestation	Number of live births plus fetal deaths	1,000
Abortion rate	Number of abortions done during a given time interval	Number of women ages 15–44 (or 49) during the same time interval	1,000

TABLE 3.4 Measures of Natality

Measure	Numerator (x)	Denominator (y)	Expressed per Number at Risk (Rate Base)
Birth rate	Number of live births reported during a given time interval	Estimated total population at mid-interval	1,000
Fertility rate	Number of live births reported during a given time interval	Estimated number of women age 15–44 (or 49) years at mid-interval	1,000
Rate of natural increase	Number of live births minus number of deaths during a given time interval	Estimated total population at mid-interval	1,000

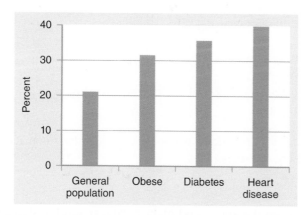

FIGURE 3.1 Arthritis prevalence among U.S. adults, 2013–2015

Data from: Barbour, K. E., Helmick, C. G., Boring, M., & Brady, T. J. Vital signs: prevalence of doctor-diagnosed arthritis and arthritis-attributable activity limitation—United States, 2013–2015.

a population (e.g., number of injuries). Lowercase letters are typically used to represent measures from a sample. A summary of some of the basic notation commonly used in statistics is shown in **TABLE 3.5**.

Greek letters are typically used to represent population characteristics (parameters). Roman letters are generally used to represent sample characteristics (statistics). For example, the parameter μ refers to the average of a given attribute in a population that is measured on a discrete or continuous scale. The statistic $\bar{x}$ is the average number of the attribute in a sample that is measured on a discrete or continuous scale.

Commonly used **measures of central location** are the arithmetic mean (average of a set of numbers), median (middle value), and mode (most frequent value). Other measures of central tendency are the midrange (sum of the lowest and highest values divided by 2) and geometric mean (central number in a geometric progression; nth root of the product of n numbers). The dispersion (spread or variation) of a distribution is the frequency and pattern of the data from the central value. Two commonly used **measures of spread** are the range

TABLE 3.5 Notation for Describing Data

Notation	Description
N	Number of observations in a population
n	Number of observations in a sample
X_1	Lowest observation in a population
X_N	Highest observation in a population
X_i	ith observation in a population
x_1	Lowest observation in a sample
x_N	Highest observation in a sample
x_i	ith observation in a sample
f_i	Frequency of the ith observation
f	Total number of observations in interval
Π	Capital Greek pi symbol, which equals the product of a sequence of numbers
Σ	Capital Greek sigma symbol, which equals the summation of a sequence of numbers

(difference between the lowest and highest values) and the standard deviation (square root of the average of the squared differences from the mean).

Numerical data involves quantitative observations where the difference between the intervals is meaningful, but there is no true definition of zero (interval), or there is a true zero (ratio) as described using certain conventional statistics. These statistics include the arithmetic mean (arithmetic average of a distribution of data); the geometric mean (nth root of the product of n observations); the median (middle value in an ordered array of data); the mode (number or value that occurs most frequently in a distribution of data); range (difference between the largest [maximum] and smallest [minimum] values of a frequency distribution); variance (mean of the squared differences of the observations from the mean); standard deviation (square root of the variance); standard error (standard deviation divided by the square root of n); and coefficient of variation (measure of relative spread in the data). Consider the following notation and equations for selected descriptive statistics (**TABLE 3.6**).

The median for numerical scaled data is obtained by (1) arranging the data in increasing or decreasing order, (2) finding the second quartile of the data $Q_2 = (n + 1)/2$, and (3) identifying the X_i value that corresponds with the second quartile. If a quartile lies on an observation (e.g., on a whole number), the value of the quartile is the value of that observation. If a quartile lies between observations, the value of the quartile is the value of the lower observation, plus the upper observation divided by 2.

TABLE 3.6 Population and Sample Equations for Selected Descriptive Measures

	Population	Sample	Sample Grouped Data
Ratio	$\dfrac{X}{Y}$	$\dfrac{x}{y}$	
Proportion	$\pi = \dfrac{X}{N}$	$p = \dfrac{x}{n}$	
Standard error of a proportion	$SE_\pi = \sqrt{\dfrac{\pi(1-\pi)}{N}}$	$SE_p = \sqrt{\dfrac{p(1-p)}{n}}$	
Arithmetic mean	$\mu = \sum\limits_{i=1}^{N} \dfrac{X_i}{N}$	$\bar{x} = \sum\limits_{i=1}^{n} \dfrac{x_i}{n}$	$\bar{X} = \sum\limits_{i=1}^{n} \dfrac{f_i X_i}{n}$
Geometric mean	$GM = \sqrt[N]{X_1 X_2 \ldots X_N}$	$GM = \sqrt[n]{\prod\limits_{i=1}^{n} x_i}$ $= \sqrt[n]{X_1 X_2 \ldots X_n}$	$GM = \sqrt[n]{\prod\limits_{i=1}^{n} X_i^{f_i}} = \sqrt[n]{X_1^{f_1} X_2^{f_2} \ldots X_n^{f_n}}$
Range	$X_N - X_1$	$x_n - x_1$	
Variance	$\sigma^2 = \dfrac{1}{N} \sum\limits_{i=1}^{N} (X_i - \mu)^2$	$s^2 = \dfrac{1}{n-1} \sum\limits_{i=1}^{n} (x_i - \bar{x})^2$	$s^2 = \dfrac{1}{\left(\sum\limits_{i=1}^{n} f_i - 1\right)} \sum\limits_{i=1}^{n} f_i (X_i - \bar{X})^2$
Standard deviation	$\sigma = \sqrt[2]{\sigma^2} = \sigma^{2/2}$	$s = \sqrt[2]{s^2} = s^{2/2}$	$s = \sqrt[2]{s^2} = s^{2/2}$
Coefficient of a variation	$\dfrac{\sigma}{\mu} \times 100$	$\dfrac{s}{x} \times 100$	

It may be of interest to identify the midrange of our data. The midrange is typically computed as $(x_1 + x_n)/2$. However, for age data, the midrange is computed as $(x_1 + x_n + 1)/2$. For example, the midrange for the age group 10–14 is $(10 + 14 + 1)/2 = 12.5$. Notice that 1 is added in order to capture those ages up to but not including 15.

A measure of central tendency that is sometimes used in epidemiology is the geometric mean. This measure is more appropriate than the arithmetic mean when exponential growth (constant proportional growth) or varying growth is involved.

Calculate the geometric mean for the data points 1, 2, 4, 8, 16.

$$GM = \sqrt[5]{1 \times 2 \times 4 \times 8 \times 16} = 4$$

In epidemiology, descriptive statistics are useful for studying the frequency, pattern, causes, and effects of health conditions (e.g., sanitation, air pollution, healthcare access), behaviors (e.g., physical activity, diet, safety precautions), and events (e.g., injury, drug abuse, suicide) in human populations.

▶ Describing Data with Graphs

A **graph** is a two-dimensional drawing showing a relationship between two sets of information or numbers. We show a relationship using a line, curve, series of bars, or other symbols in a simple, compact format. Graphs can help clarify a public health problem by identifying patterns, trends, aberrations, similarities, and differences in data. They are helpful for describing and communicating health-related states or events according to person, place, and time. The building blocks of graphs are numbers, ratios, proportions, or rates. Some common graphical methods that are used for displaying data are presented in **TABLE 3.7**.

TABLE 3.7 Graphs for Describing Data

Type of Graph	When to Use
Arithmetic-scale line graph (example: Figure 2.4)	Line graphs are used mostly for data plotted against time. An arithmetic graph has equal quantities along the y-axis. An arithmetic graph shows actual changes in the magnitude of the number or rate of a health-related state or event across time.
Logarithmic-scale line graph (example: Figure 2.3)	The y-axis is changed to a logarithmic scale. In other words, the axis is divided into cycles, with each being 10 times greater than the previous cycle. The focus is on the rate of change. A straight line reflects a constant rate of change.
Simple bar chart (example: Figure 1.1)	A visual display of the magnitude of the different categories of a single variable, with each category or value of the variable represented by a bar.
Histogram (example: Figures 1.3, 1.4)	A graphic representation of the frequency distribution of a variable. Rectangles are drawn so that their bases lie on a linear scale representing different intervals, and their heights are proportional to the frequencies of the values within each of the intervals.
Spot map (e.g., John Snow's spot map)	A map that indicates the location of each case of a rare health-related state or event by a place that is potentially relevant to the health event being investigated, such as where each case lived or worked.
Area map (e.g., cancer rates by state and county)	A map that indicates the number or rate of a health-related state or event by place, using different colors or shadings to represent the various levels of the disease, event, behavior, or condition.
Scatter plot (**FIGURE 3.2**)	This graph is a useful summary of the association between two numerical variables. It is usually drawn before calculating a linear correlation coefficient or fitting a regression line, because these statistics assume a linear relationship in the data. It provides a good visual picture of the relationship between the two variables and aids in the interpretation of the correlation coefficient or regression model.
Population pyramid	A graphical illustration that shows the distribution of age groups in a population for males and females.

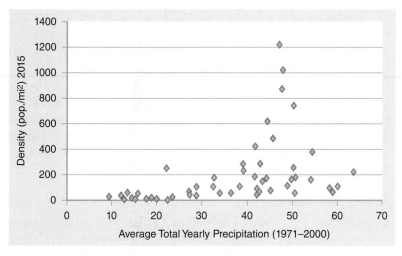

FIGURE 3.2 Scatter plot showing the relationship between population density and annual precipitation

Data from https://en.wikipedia.org/wiki/List_of_U.S._states_and_territories_by_population_density#cite_note-PopEstUS-1; https://www.currentresults.com/Weather/US/average-annual-state-precipitation.php.

Summary

1. Descriptive statistics in epidemiology are useful for studying the frequency, pattern, causes, and effects of health conditions (e.g., sanitation, air pollution, healthcare access), behaviors (e.g., physical activity, diet, safety precautions), and events (e.g., injury, drug abuse, suicide) in human populations.

2. Statistics is the science of data, a branch of mathematics that involves collecting, classifying, summarizing, organizing, analyzing, and interpreting data. The four general areas of statistics are: descriptive, probability, inferential, and statistical techniques.

3. The scale of measurement represents the precision wherein an attribute is measured. The three scales of measurement used in epidemiology are nominal, ordinal, and numerical. Nominal data is comprised of qualitative or categorical observations with no inherent ordering. Ordinal data is also comprised of qualitative or categorical observations, but with an inherent ordering. Numerical data is comprised of quantitative observations that may be discrete or continuous. Discrete data can only take values that you can count, and continuous data can take on any value within a range.

4. A frequency distribution is a tabular summary of a set of data that shows the frequency or number of data items that fall into each of several distinct classes. A frequency distribution is also known as a "frequency table." The relative frequency of a category is the frequency of that category divided by the total number of observations.

5. A ratio is the number of observations with the characteristic of interest divided by the number without the characteristic of interest. A proportion is the number of observations with the characteristic of interest divided by the total number of observations. A rate is a number of cases of a particular outcome divided by the size of the at-risk population in that time period, multiplied by a base (e.g., 100, 1,000, 10,000, or 100,000).

6. To summarize and describe numerical scale data, we use measures of central location (e.g., arithmetic mean, median, mode, midrange, geometric mean) and dispersion (e.g., range, standard deviation, variance, coefficient of variation).

7. A graph is a two-dimensional drawing showing a relationship between two sets of information or numbers. Graphs can help clarify a public health problem by identifying patterns, trends, aberrations, similarities, and differences in data. The building blocks of graphs are numbers, ratios, proportions, and rates.

Computer Application

1. Open the Excel workbook Application 3.1.xlsx. Within the spreadsheet is a frequency distribution table. Put the cursor over cells in the D, E, and F columns to see how the table was generated. Delete the values in these cells and duplicate them on your own.

2. Open the Excel workbook Application 3.2.xlsx. Put your cursor over each of the cells in Column E to see how the answers were obtained using Excel.

3. Open the Excel workbook Application 3.3.xlsx. Refer to the data in A2 through A22. Compute the mean, median, range, and variance for the sample, the standard deviation for the sample, and the coefficient of variation. Refer to the data in D2 through D6 and compute the geometric mean. Refer to the data in cells G2 through H6 and compute the geometric mean. Refer to the data in cells K2 through K7 and compute the middle age in each age range.

4. Open Epi Info and select CLASSIC. In this tab, go to the data folder on the left side of the screen and select Read. We want to import data from an Excel workbook.[1] Under Database Type, select Microsoft Excel 2007 Workbook (.xlsx). Then select Browse and identify Application 3.4.xlsx.

    Under Data Source Explorer, select Sheet1$ and then click OK. In the Output screen will appear:

    Current Data Source: F:\Application 3.4.xlsx *Record Count:* 674 *(Deleted Records Excluded) Date:* 7/14/2017 10:54:13 AM

    In the Program Editor, you will see:

    READ {F:\Application 3.4.xlsx}

    To view the data set, go to the Statistics folder on the left side of the screen and select List, and then under Variables, enter * (to see the data for all the variables) and click OK. Now, go to Frequencies and select Frequency of Intervention. This will show the frequency distribution table for those in and not in the intervention at baseline. There are 170 in the control group and 167 in the intervention group. Now create a table of the intervention status by gender. Go to Tables, and for the Exposure Variable, select the Group variable; for the Outcome Variable, select Sex. This shows us that there are 71.8% females in the intervention group and 73.1% females in the control group. In the Single Table Analysis output, there are several statistics that we will discuss later in the book.

    Now we will explore the mean Age for those in the intervention versus the control group. Go to Means, enter Mean of Age, and enter Stratify by Group. The results will show that the mean age is very similar between the groups (50.39 vs. 50.83).

You can also compare means by choosing Summarize. Under Aggregate, select Average. Under Variable, select Age. Under Group By, select Group. Under Into Variable, type Age and select Apply. Under Output to Table, type A. Then click OK. In a similar way, obtain the means for BMI, Body Fat, Health Test, and Total Steps (week).

Finally, we will create a graph showing the number of males and females in the intervention and control groups. Select Graph and then under Graph Type, select Bar. Select Sex as the Main Variable, and type Sex as the Independent Axis Label. For the Dependent Axis Label, type Number. Under Show Value of, select Count. Under Series Bar of Each Value of, select Group. For Title, type "Sex according to group status."

5. Create your own area map by going to the CDC homepage and searching for "WISQARS™ Tutorials: Fatal Injury Mapping."

6. To create a population pyramid, go to census.gov and search for "International Programs Information Gateway."

Under Select Report, highlight and click Population Pyramid Graph. Under Select up to 25 Years, click 2018. Then choose a country of interest and click Submit. The distribution of males and females across the age span is then represented.

Reference

1. Aldana, S. G., Greenlaw, R. L., Diehl, H. A., Salberg, A., Merrill, R. M., & Ohmine, S. (2005). The effects of a worksite chronic disease prevention program. *Journal of Occupational Environmental Medicine, 47(6)*, 558–564.

Practice Problems

3.1

Complete the following frequency distribution table for the number of children born to 50 women. Round your answer to the nearest hundredth.

Number of Children	Frequency	Relative Frequency	Cumulative Frequency	Cumulative Relative Frequency
0	8			
1	11			
2	14			
3	8			
4	5			
5+	4			

What percentage of women had fewer than three children? _____

What percentage of women had two or three children? _____

3.2

For a rate base of 100,000, what is z? _____

3.3

In a city of 4,386 people, 126 attended a potluck dinner. Among those attending the dinner, within 4 hours some began to experience diarrhea and abdominal distress. Between 6–72 hours following the dinner, 78 individuals experienced symptoms that included acute diarrhea, abdominal pain, fever, and vomiting. These symptoms and the incubation period were consistent with the disease salmonella. What was the attack rate? Round your answer to the nearest tenth.

_____

3.4

Refer to Problem 3.3. If 65% of the people who attended the dinner were female and their rate of illness was 64.6 per 100, how many females became ill?

_____

3.5

Suppose that 20 children in a daycare center came down with a strain of influenza. A total of 480 people lived in the households where these cases resided. In those households, there were a total of 120 cases. What was the primary attack rate? Express your answer with the rate base.

_____

3.6

Refer to problem 3.5. What is the secondary attack rate? Express your answer using an appropriate rate base and to the nearest tenth.

_____

3.7

The prevalence of doctor-diagnosed arthritis among adults living in the United States on January 1, 2018, was 55.2 million. The adult population was 240,000,000. What was the point prevalence proportion for this disease? Express your answer as a percent.

_____%

3.8

Suppose that in the general adult population, the prevalence of arthritis is 23%. For those who are obese, it is 34.8% higher; for those who have high blood pressure, it is 91.3% higher; for those who have diabetes, it is 104.3% higher; and for those who have heart disease, it is 113.0% higher. What is the estimated point prevalence proportion (per 100) of arthritis among adults living in the United States on January 1, 2018, for each of these diseases? Express your answer as a percent.

Obesity: _____%

High blood pressure: _____%

Diabetes: _____%

Heart disease: _____%

3.9

Statistics for a Hypothetical Population, July 1 through June 30

Total 1-year population	170,000
Population of women 15–49	45,000
Population of 55 years of age and older	46,000
Number of live births	3,250
Number of fetal deaths after 20 weeks' gestation	65
Number of maternal deaths	5
Total deaths	1,500
Number of infant deaths from birth through 27 days	50
Number of infant deaths between 28 and 364 days of age	40
Number of infant deaths between 0 and 1 year of age	90
Number of deaths of persons 55 years of age and older	850
Number of deaths from heart disease	140
Number of deaths from cancer	80
Number of deaths from stroke	60
Number of deaths from accidents	45
Number of deaths from cancer in persons 55 years of age and older	42
Number of persons diagnosed with heart disease	530
Number of persons diagnosed with high blood pressure, arteriosclerosis, or atherosclerosis	1,500
Number of abortions	2,480

Calculate the following using an appropriate rate base with 0 places after the decimal:

1. Crude mortality rate	
2. Maternal mortality rate	
3. Infant mortality rate	
4. Neonatal mortality rate	
5. Post-neonatal mortality rate	
6. Fetal death rate	
7. Fertility rate	
8. Age-specific mortality rate for persons 55 years of age and older	
9. Cause-specific mortality rate for heart disease	
10. Cause-specific mortality rate for stroke	
11. Proportional mortality ratio for cancer among persons 55 years of age and older	
12. Death-to-case ratio for heart disease	
13. Abortion rate	
14. Rate of natural increase	

3.10

For the following data that consists of the number of children for 21 women, calculate the arithmetic mean _____, median _____, range _____, variance _____ , standard deviation _____, standard error _____, and coefficient of variation _____. Round your answers to the nearest hundredth.

Children	Number
0	5
1	5
2	4
3	3
4	3
5	1

3.11

Calculate the geometric mean (rounding to the nearest hundredth) for the following data:

X	f
1	1
2	2
4	4
8	6
16	3

3.12

The death rate for diabetes mellitus (per 100,000) is 50, 75, 100, 150, and 210 in the age groups 60–64, 65–69, 70–74, 75–79, and 80–84, respectively. What is the geometric mean for these data? Round your answer to the nearest tenth.

3.13

Calculate the midrange for each of the following age groups. Round your answer to the nearest tenth.

0–4	
5–9	
10–14	
15–19	
20–24	
25–29	

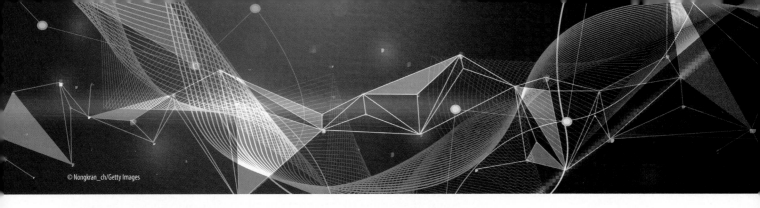

CHAPTER 4
Probability in Epidemiology

Probability is the second major topic in the area of statistics. It indicates how likely it is that something will happen. It provides a basis for evaluating the reliability of the conclusions we reach and the inferences we make when applying statistical techniques to the collection, analysis, and interpretation of data. In epidemiology, probability is used to indicate the likelihood of each outcome of a random variable (i.e., a variable whose numerical value is determined by a chance mechanism), the likelihood that an event will occur given a previous event, the representativeness of a sample, the likelihood that a parameter lies within a range around a statistic, and the likelihood that a result is due to chance.

The purpose of this chapter is to introduce you to probability concepts, probability sampling, probability distribution, point estimates and confidence intervals, and the *p*-value.

▶ Probability Concepts

Probability is a familiar concept. The personal notion of probability is subjective because it is based on opinion and past experience, rather than on formal calculations. **Subjective probability** is influenced by personal judgment as to whether a given event will occur. For example, the probability that you are going to be late for work is greater if you do not set your alarm. Alternatively, **objective probability** is the likelihood of the outcome of any event based on repeated random experiments or measurements rather than subjective assessment. An **event** is one or more outcomes of an experiment. Two events are dependent if the occurrence of the first event affects the occurrence of the second event, thereby changing the probability. For example, the probability of contracting a disease depends on the probability of being exposed to a given risk factor or whether you were vaccinated for the disease. Two events are independent if the probability of one event does not influence the probability of another event. For example, blood type is independent of Rhesus (Rh) factor (an inherited protein on the surface of red blood cells).

In the context of objective probability, the term "experiment" refers to any planned process of data collection. An **experiment** is an operation that consists of a number of independent trials (replications of experiments) under stable conditions and results in any one of a set of outcomes; it is an operation that produces observations or measurements. The actual outcome cannot be predicted with certainty. For example, an experiment may consist of treating AIDS patients with a new drug and evaluating whether they respond favorably. The set of all possible outcomes of an experiment is referred to as the **sample space**. Because the sample space S contains all possible outcomes of the experiment, the probability of S is equal to 1.

$$P(S) = 1$$

Within a sample space there is usually a smaller set of outcomes, which we call "events". The probability of an event reflects the result of an experiment; it is the proportion of times that the event occurs over the total number of repetitions of the experiment. The probability of a given event A is

$$0 \leq P(A) \leq 1$$

We can express probabilities as proportions in the range 0 to 1 or as percentages in the range 0% to 100%. For the data appearing in **TABLE 4.1**, the sample space is the set of 12 mutually exclusive events. Note that in probability theory, two events are mutually exclusive (or disjoint) if the occurrence of one precludes the occurrence of another. For example, having one stage of a cancer precludes you from having another stage of the cancer; that is, you cannot have multiple stages of cancer at the same time. To illustrate, the probability of distant-stage disease is 0.154. This means that the probability of having either local- or regional-stage disease is $1 - 0.154 = 0.846$. This latter expression is the complement of distant-stage disease.

Sometimes we are interested in knowing the probability that an event will not happen. This is called a **complementary event**. The probability of a complementary event may be found as 1 minus the probability of the primary event. If $\bar{A}$ is the complement of event A, then

TABLE 4.1 Sample Space for Cervical Cancer in the United States According to Tumor Stage at Diagnosis and Race, 2011–2013

Stage	Probabilities				
	White	Black	American Indian or Alaska Native	Asian or Pacific Islander	Total
Localized	0.355	0.052	0.005	0.042	0.454
Regional	0.285	0.064	0.004	0.039	0.392
Distant	0.111	0.025	0.003	0.015	0.154
Total	0.751	0.141	0.012	0.096	1.000

Data from: Surveillance, Epidemiology, and End Results (SEER) Program (www.seer.cancer.gov) SEER*Stat Database: Incidence—SEER 18 Regs Research Data + Hurricane Katrina Impacted Louisiana Cases, November 2015 Submission (2000–2013) <Katrina/Rita Population Adjustment>—Linked to County Attributes, Total U.S., 1969–2014 Counties, National Cancer Institute, DCCPS, Surveillance Research Program, Surveillance Systems Branch, released April 2016, based on the November 2015 submission.

$$P(\bar{A}) = 1 - P(A)$$

We are also often interested in knowing the probability of an event "given" or "conditional" on the occurrence of another event. Using the vertical line | to mean "given," we can mathematically express the probability of one event given another as

$$P(A|B) = \frac{P(A \text{ and } B)}{P(B)} \quad \text{where } P(A) > 0$$

To illustrate, the probability of having distant-stage disease if you are black is

$$P(\text{Local stage}|\text{Black}) = \frac{0.025}{0.141} = 0.177$$

Rule for Addition of Probabilities of Mutually Exclusive Events
If events A and B are mutually exclusive, then
$$P(A \text{ or } B) = P(A) + P(B)$$

To illustrate, the probability of regional or distant-stage cervical cancer is

$$P(\text{Regional stage or Distant}) = P(\text{Regional stage}) + P(\text{Distant stage})$$
$$= 0.392 + 0.154 = 0.546$$

The addition rule also applies for more than two mutually exclusive events. In many situations, events are not mutually exclusive. The rule of probabilities that are not mutually exclusive are presented in the following box.

Rule for Probabilities That Are Not Mutually Exclusive Events
If events A and B are not mutually exclusive, then
$$P(A \text{ or } B) = P(A) + P(B) - P(A \text{ and } B)$$

The probability of having distant-stage cervical cancer and being black is

$$P(\text{Distant stage or Black}) = P(\text{Distant stage}) + P(\text{Black})$$
$$- P(\text{Distant stage and Black})$$
$$= 0.154 + 0.141 - 0.025$$
$$= 0.27$$

A conditional probability that is commonly applied in epidemiology involves the probability of disease given a specific exposure. For example, if 35% of adults in the United States are obese, and 11% have arthritis and are obese, what is the probability of arthritis among obese individuals?

$$P(\text{Arthritis}|\text{Obese}) = \frac{P(\text{Arthritis and Obese})}{P(\text{Obese})} = \frac{0.11}{0.35} = 0.31$$

Two events A and B are statistically independent if $P(A | B) = P(A)$; i.e., $P(A \text{ and } B) = P(A) \times P(B)$. The occurrence of event B gives no information about the probability of event A.

$$P(\text{Heart disease}) = 0.25$$

$$P(\text{Coffee}) = 0.40$$

$$P(\text{Heart disease and Coffee}) = 0.10$$

Then, $P(\text{Heart disease}|\text{Coffee}) = \dfrac{P(\text{Heart disease and Coffee})}{P(\text{Coffee})} = \dfrac{0.10}{0.40} = 0.25$

	Heart Disease	**No Heart Disease**	
Coffee	0.10	0.30	.40
No coffee	0.15	0.45	.60
	0.25	0.75	1.00

So, the occurrence of coffee drinking gives no information about the probability of heart disease.

In general, if the events A and B are statistically independent, then the ratio of $P(A|B)$ divided by $P(A|\bar{B})$ equals 1. For example, in the previous problem

$$\frac{P(A|B)}{P(A|\bar{B})} = \frac{0.25}{0.25} = 1; \text{No association}$$

If A and B are not independent

$$\frac{P(A|B)}{P(A|\bar{B})} > 1; \text{Positive association}$$

$$\frac{P(A|B)}{P(A|\bar{B})} < 1; \text{Negative association}$$

Conditional probability is also commonly used in epidemiology to assess the validity of a test. In this situation, we are interested in determining how well the test actually measures what it is supposed to measure. In **TABLE 4.2**, the true disease status (present or not present) is represented at the top of the table, and the left side represents the test result (positive or negative).

True positive (TP) means a person has the disease and they test positive; true negative (TN) means a person does not have the disease and they test negative; false positive (FP) means a person does not have the disease but they test positive; false negative (FN) means a person has the disease but they test negative. Five measures of validity for evaluating a test are as follows:

$$P(+ \mid D) = P\left(\frac{TP}{TP + FN}\right) = \text{Sensitivity}$$

$$P(- \mid \bar{D}) = P\left(\frac{TN}{FP + TN}\right) = \text{Specificity}$$

$$P(D \mid +) = P\left(\frac{TP}{TP + FP}\right) = \text{Predictive value positive}$$

$$P(\bar{D} \mid -) = P\left(\frac{TN}{TN + FN}\right) = \text{Predictive value negative}$$

$$P(\text{Correct result} \mid \text{All possible results}) = P\left(\frac{TP + TN}{TP + TN + FP + FN}\right)$$
$$= \text{Overall accuracy}$$

TABLE 4.2 Test Results and True Disease Status

Test Result	True Disease Status	
	Disease (D)	No Disease ($\bar{D}$)
Positive (+)	TP	FP
Negative (−)	FN	TN
	TP + FN	FP + TN

TABLE 4.3 Prostate-Specific Antigen Screening for Prostate Cancer

Test Result	True Prostate Cancer Status	
	Present	Not Present
PSA ≥ 4	110	786
PSA < 4	21	524
	131	1,310

A valid screening test minimizes the threat of a false positive test—which may cause unnecessary stress, anxiety, and treatment—and a false negative test, which may cause an individual to not receive needed treatment.

A common screening test for prostate cancer is a blood test that measures prostate-specific antigen (PSA) in the blood (**TABLE 4.3**). Assume that a PSA score of at least 4 is a positive test.

What is the sensitivity of the test?

$$\text{Sensitivity} = \frac{110}{131} = 0.84$$

What is the specificity of the test?

$$\text{Specificity} = \frac{524}{1,310} = 0.40$$

Of those with a positive test, what proportion has prostate cancer?

$$\text{Predictive value positive} = \frac{\text{TP}}{\text{TP} + \text{FP}} = 0.12$$

Of those with a negative test, what proportion does not have prostate cancer?

$$\text{Predictive value negative} = \frac{\text{TN}}{\text{FN} + \text{TN}} = 0.96$$

What is the overall accuracy of the test?

$$\text{Overall accuracy} = \frac{110 + 524}{110 + 786 + 21 + 524} = 0.44$$

When the prior probability of a disease is known, then we use a more complicated formula for predictive value positive and predictive value negative, which utilizes Bayes' Theorem. This formula will not be presented in this book, but it is readily available in many introductory epidemiology books.

▶ Probability Sampling

A **sample** is a subset of items that have been selected from the population. There are a number of reasons we may study a sample instead of a population. When the population is large, a sample can be studied more quickly, less expensively, and more accurately. In many situations, it may be impossible to access an entire population.

A probability sampling method involves a sample with some form of random selection wherein the different units in the population have an equal probability of being selected. Probability methods can be employed to make probability statements about observations and to estimate the error in the resulting statistics. The best way to obtain a sample wherein the results produce valid inferences to the larger population is to use probability samples. Common probability sampling methods that are based on a random process include simple random sampling, systematic sampling, stratified sampling, and cluster sampling. Basic terms used in these probability methods are

N = number of cases in the sampling frame

n = number of cases in the sample

$\left(\dfrac{N}{n} \right)$ = number of combinations of size n from N

$f = n/N$ = the sampling fraction

$$\left(\frac{N}{n} \right) = \frac{N!}{n!} = \frac{N(N-1)\ldots(N-N+1)}{n(n-1)\ldots(n-n+1)}$$

If $N = 3$ and $n = 2$, then

$$\left(\frac{3}{2} \right) = \frac{3!}{2!} = \frac{3(3-1)(3-3+1)}{2(2-1)(2-2+1)} = \frac{6}{2} = 3$$

This means in a population of 3, there are 3 ways to take a sample of 2; that is, persons 1 and 2, persons 2 and 3, and persons 1 and 3.

A **simple random sample** is a sample that is selected from a finite population in such a way that all samples of the same size have the same probability of being chosen. To randomly select a sample from a population, we need a sampling frame, which is a list that contains every member of the population. Suppose a population of interest has 1000 people and we wish to take a random sample of 100. A unique number will be required for each person in the population, from 1 to 1000. Then, using a random number generator, we can select our 100 numbers. In an Excel workbook, we can calculate random numbers. In the worksheet, put the cursor in any cell, then type = RANDBETWEEN(Bottom number, Top number) and press the Enter key. This will give a random number in the range specified. We can copy this formula and paste it over the number of cells for which we are interested in obtaining random numbers.

A **systematic sample** is one where every kth item is selected. First, we number the population from 1 to N; second, we decide on the appropriate sample size n; third, the interval size is obtained by dividing the number of items in the **sampling frame** (a population list from which items or people are sampled) by the desired sample size $k = N/n$; fourth, we randomly select an integer between 1 and k; and fifth, we take every kth unit. Systematic sampling should only be used when a cyclic repetition is not inherent in the sampling frame.

A **stratified random sample** (also called "proportional" or "quota" random sampling) involves dividing the population into non-overlapping subgroups (strata), $N_1 + N_2 + \cdots + N_i = N$, and then taking a simple random sample of $f = n/N$ in each subgroup (e.g., age, gender, socioeconomic status, religion, nationality, educational attainment). This sampling approach is more common in epidemiology than in clinical studies because clusters are commonly based on geographic areas (e.g., a sample for a hospital survey taken in a state may be selected by using census tracts as clusters, with a sample then taken of hospitals in each census tract). Stratified random sampling assures that key subgroups of the population are represented, thus allowing you to be able to say something about these groups in your analysis. It also provides more statistical precision than simple random sampling if the strata are homogeneous.

If we wanted to sample 100 from a population of 1000, and 70% are white, 10% are black, 10% are Hispanic, and 10% are Asian, then a random sample of the population would result in about 70 whites, 10 blacks, 10 Hispanics, and 10 Asians. However, if 25 per group are needed to make meaningful comparisons among the racial or ethnic groups, the corresponding sampling fractions would be $25/700 = 0.036$ (or 3.6%) for whites, $25/100 = .25$ (or 25%) for blacks, $25/100 = .25$ (or 25%) for Hispanics, and $25/100 = .25$ (or 25%) for Asians.

A challenge with random sampling occurs when the population of interest is dispersed over a large geographic area. Hence, a sample would involve covering a lot of ground geographically. A more efficient approach would be to conduct a cluster sample. The steps to conducting a cluster sample are:

1. Divide the population into clusters.
2. Randomly sample the clusters.
3. Measure all the units within the sampled clusters.

Thus, a **cluster sample** involves a form of probability sample where respondents are drawn from a random sample of mutually exclusive groups (clusters) within a total population. Cluster sampling may be less expensive and more convenient than simple random sampling. For example, suppose you want to survey elderly people in a specific region. If you conducted a random sample of all these individuals, you might have to visit all senior care centers in the region to interview the entire sample. With cluster sampling, we could first select the senior care centers to be included in the sample, and then select individuals within each of the facilities. That would probably reduce the number of facilities we would need to visit and, consequently, reduce the cost of data collection. In addition, visiting a smaller number of facilities could also improve the quality of data collection.

▶ Probability Distribution

A discrete variable is a variable that involves countable values, such as the number of visits to an emergency room on a given day. The variable is random if the sum of the probabilities is equal to 1. A discrete distribution describes the probability of occurrence for each value of the discrete random variable. Probabilities are given by a probability distribution function $P(X = x)$, graphically represented by the height of the bars in a bar graph. For example, let X represent the number of children among a group of women. The $P(X = 0)$ means

TABLE 4.4 Discrete Probability Distribution for Number of Children						
x	0	1	2	3	4	5+
P(X = x)	2/35	8/35	13/35	7/35	3/35	2/35

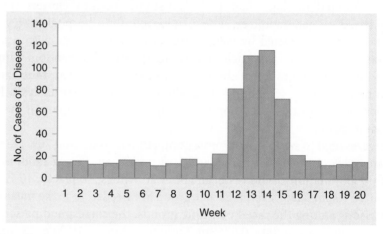

FIGURE 4.1 Endemic versus epidemic

the probability of no children. Consider the discrete probability distribution in **TABLE 4.4**.

The cumulative distribution function of a discrete random variable X is the function $F(t)$, which represents the probability that X is less than or equal to t:

$$F(T) = P(X \leq t)$$

For example,

$$P(X \leq 2) = \frac{2}{35} + \frac{8}{35} + \frac{13}{35} = \frac{23}{35} = 0.657$$

Time is a continuous variable, but if we classify time according to certain units, like days, weeks, and years, where we can list the values it can take on, we have made the variable discrete. For example, assume a set of data measured by weeks (**FIGURE 4.1**). This graph shows that endemic (expected) levels of a disease tend to range from 12 to 18 in any given week, except weeks 12 through 15, wherein the disease is at epidemic (unexpected) levels.

A continuous random variable is a random variable that has infinitely many values, such as time. A random variable that measures time is continuous because there is an infinite number of possible times. A continuous distribution describes probabilities associated with the possible values of a continuous random variable. The equation that describes a continuous probability distribution is called a "probability density function." Probability density functions satisfy certain conditions:

1. The random variable Y is a function of X; $y = f(x)$.
2. $y \geq 0$ for all values of x.
3. The total area under the probability density function curve is equal to 1.

For those who have studied calculus, finding the area under a probability density curve involves the use of integration. For example, the area between a and b below the probability density curve is expressed as

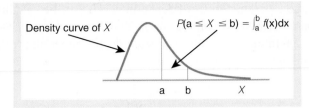

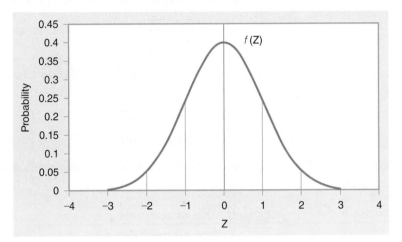

FIGURE 4.2 Standard normal curve

In statistics, the normal distribution is a very commonly used continuous probability distribution. The simplest type of normal distribution is the standard normal distribution, where $\mu = 0$ and $\sigma = 1$, and the probability density function is

$$f(x) = \frac{e^{-(1/2)x^2}}{\sqrt{2\pi}}$$

This function is symmetric around 0, and the total area under the curve $f(x)$ equals 1 (**FIGURE 4.2**).

We will revisit this probability density function later when we talk about hypothesis testing.

▶ Point Estimates and Confidence Intervals

The purpose of sampling from a population is to construct a sample quantity that will estimate an unknown population value called a **parameter**. This sample quantity is called an **estimator**, which is a random variable or a sample statistic that is used to estimate an unknown population parameter. The actual numerical value obtained for an estimator is called an **estimate**, or **point estimate**. For example, if $x_1,\ldots, x_n$ is a random sample of size n from $f(X)$, with $E(X) = \mu$ and $Var(X) = \sigma^2$, then we can estimate the population mean μ using the sample mean $\bar{x}$ and the population variance σ^2 using the sample variance s^2.

Along with a point estimate, we are interested in estimating an interval that indicates a range in which the parameter is likely to fall. A confidence interval defines an upper limit and a lower limit with an associated probability. The probability statement is about the confidence interval rather than the population parameter. A confidence interval based on a single sample indicates that there is a certain probability (or percent age, usually 95%) that the derived confidence interval from a future assessment of the data will contain the true value of the population parameter. Confidence intervals can be calculated for any population parameter. If the sample size is 30 or more, then a 95% confidence interval uses 1.96 in its calculation. For example, the equation for the 95% confidence interval of the population mean is

$$\bar{x} \pm 1.96 \frac{s}{\sqrt{n}}$$

The equation for the 95% confidence interval of the population proportion is

$$p \pm 1.96 \sqrt{\frac{p(1-p)}{n}}$$

The equation for the 95% confidence interval of the population attack rate is given as

$$\text{Rate} \pm 1.96 \sqrt{\frac{\text{Rate}(1 - \text{Rate})}{\text{Population at risk}}}$$

The equation for the 95% confidence interval of the population person-time rate is given as

$$\text{Rate} \pm 1.96 \sqrt{\frac{\text{No. of new cases}}{(\text{Person-time at risk})^2}}$$

In general, confidence intervals are used to indicate the precision of any statistical measure based on a sample.

▶ *p*-Value

When samples are involved, statistical measures obtained from units of interest may vary from sample to sample. As a result, a statistical finding may be the result of chance: the "luck of the draw." That is, it is possible that the selected sample is not representative of the population, merely because of bad luck. To minimize this risk, we use probability sampling, as discussed previously, from a sufficiently large sample size. As the sample size increases, the risk of misrepresentation decreases. The determination of appropriate sample sizes is based on equations that take into account certain expectations that will be discussed in biostatistics and more advanced epidemiology classes.

The *p*-value is a probability that ranges from 0 to 1 and provides a means for evaluating the role of chance. For example, suppose a statistical measure of association indicates a negative relationship between sleep and workplace injuries. A corresponding *p*-value for the statistical measure is 0.02, which says there is a small probability that the finding is due to chance, merely 2%. The **p-value** is defined as the probability of obtaining an effect at least as large as the one in your sample data, given that the null hypothesis is true; To fully understand the *p*-value, we first need to introduce you to hypothesis testing. Hypothesis testing involves first specifying what we think is happening on the population level, and then evaluating this supposition based on results from sampled data. In other words, we attempt to infer from sample data what we think might exist in the population. Inferential statistics is used to make judgments about the probability that an estimated result is real and not due to chance. The role of the *p*-value in hypothesis testing will be explained more fully in the next chapter.

Summary

1. In epidemiology, probability is used to indicate the likelihood of each outcome of a random variable, the likelihood that an event will occur given a previous event, the representativeness of a sample, the likelihood that a parameter lies within a range around a statistic, and the likelihood that a result is due to chance.

2. Subjective probability is influenced by personal judgment as to whether a given event will occur. For example, the probability that I am going to perform poorly in my piano recital is greater if I do not practice. Objective probability is the likelihood of the outcome of any event based upon repeated random experiments or measurements rather than on subjective assessment.

3. Two events are independent if the probability of one event does not influence the probability of another event.

4. An experiment is an operation that consists of a number of independent trials (replications of experiments) under stable conditions and that results in any one of a set of outcomes.

5. The set of all possible outcomes of an experiment is referred to as the "sample space."

6. Two events are mutually exclusive (or disjoint) if the occurrence of one precludes the occurrence of another. If events A and B are mutually exclusive, then $P(A \text{ or } B) = P(A) + P(B)$. If events A and B are not mutually exclusive, then $P(A \text{ or } B) = P(A) + P(B) - P(A \text{ and } B)$.

7. A valid screening test minimizes the threat of a false positive test—which may cause unnecessary stress, anxiety, and treatment—and a false negative test, which may cause an individual to forgo needed treatment.

8. A sample is a subset of items that have been selected from the population. A probability sample involves taking a sample with some form of random selection in which the different units in the population have an equal probability of being selected. Common probability sampling methods that are based on a random process include simple random sampling, systematic sampling, stratified sampling, and cluster sampling.

9. A discrete distribution describes the probability of occurrence for each value of the discrete random variable.

10. A continuous distribution describes probabilities associated with the possible values of a continuous random variable.

11. A sample quantity used to estimate an unknown population value is called an "estimator." The actual numerical value obtained for an estimator is called an "estimate," or "point estimate."

12. A confidence interval defines an upper limit and a lower limit with an associated probability. The probability statement is about the confidence interval rather than the population parameter. A confidence interval based on a single sample indicates that there is a certain probability (or percentage, usually 95%) that the derived confidence interval from a future assessment of the data will contain the true value of the population parameter.

13. The p-value is the probability that an effect as large or larger than that observed in a particular study could have occurred by chance alone, given that the null hypothesis is true.

Computer Application

1. Open the Excel workbook Application 4.1.xlsx. Answer the probability concept questions using Excel.

2. Open the Excel workbook Application 4.2.xlsx. Answer the probability sampling questions using Excel.

3. Open the Excel workbook Application 4.3.xlsx. Answer the probability distribution and confidence interval questions using Excel.

4. Start Epi Info 7 and select STATCALC. Now select POISSON (RARE EVENT VS. STANDARD). In the injury exercise, there were 10 injuries. Enter 10 in the Observed # of events cell. Now suppose that on average, there are 5 injuries that occur during the same period of follow-up. Enter 5 in the Expected # of events cell. Based on past experience, what is the probability of there being 10 or more injuries?

Practice Problems

4.1

Refer to Table 4.1 in the text. What is the probability of being staged with localized disease?

_____

4.2

Refer to Table 4.1 in the text. What is the complement of localized cervical cancer?

_____

4.3

Refer to Table 4.1 in the text. Among cervical cancer patients, what is the probability of locally staged disease given that the racial group is white? Black? American Indian or Alaska Native? Asian or Pacific Islander? Round your answers to the nearest thousandth.

White _____

Black _____

American Indian/Alaska Native _____

Asian/Pacific Islander _____

4.4

Refer to Table 4.1 in the text. What is the probability of local- or regional-stage cervical cancer?

_____

4.5

Refer to Table 4.1 in the text. What is the probability of having local-stage cervical cancer and being white?

_____

4.6

Refer to the data in the following table. What is the probability of heart disease, smoking, smoking and heart disease, heart disease for a smoker? Round your answers to the nearest hundredth.

	Heart Disease	No Heart Disease	
Smoker	0.05	0.15	.20
Nonsmoker	0.15	0.65	.80
	0.2	0.8	1.00

Heart disease: _____

Smoking: _____

Smoking and heart disease: _____

Heart disease for a smoker: _____

4.7

Using the data in Table 4.1 in the text, show whether diagnosis with distant staged cervical cancer is associated with being black versus white, American Indian/Alaska Native versus white, and Asian or Pacific Islander versus white. Round your answers to the nearest hundredth.

Black versus white: _____

American Indian/Alaska Native versus white: _____

Asian or Pacific Islander versus white: _____

For problems 4.8–4.12, refer to the following table.

Test Results According to Disease Status

	Disease	
Test Result	Yes	No
+	67	155
−	12	628
	79	783

4.8

What is the sensitivity of the test?

_____

4.9

What is the specificity of the test?

_____

4.10

Of those with a positive test, what proportion has prostate cancer?

_____

4.11

Of those with a negative test, what proportion does not have prostate cancer?

_____

4.12

What is the overall accuracy of the test?

_____

4.13

If $N = 4$ and $n = 3$, how many samples are possible?

_____

4.14

What is the sampling fraction when $n = 100$ and $N = 1000$?

_____

4.15

How would you proceed with a systematic sample based on a desired sample size of 100 from a population of size 1000?

4.16

In the context of sampling, what is the difference between strata and clusters?

4.17

Refer to Table 4.4 in the text. What is the probability of having one child? Round your answer to the nearest thousandth.

4.18

Refer to Table 4.4 in the text. What is the probability of having no more than three children? Round your answer to the nearest thousandth.

4.19

Calculate the 95% confidence interval for the mean weight of a population of students, based on a sample size of 50, a sample mean ($\bar{x}$) of 120, and a standard deviation (which is a measure of variability in our sample), of 25. Round your answer to the nearest tenth.

4.20

Calculate the 95% confidence interval for the proportion of obese individuals in a population of students, based on a sample size of 100 and a sample proportion (p) of 0.2. Round your answer to the nearest hundredth.

4.21

Calculate the 95% confidence interval for the rate of female breast cancer, based on a sample size of 446,686 and a sample rate of 0.00142. Express your answer per 100,000.

4.22

Calculate the 95% confidence interval for the person-time rate of injury, based on 10 injuries occurring over 16,800 hours worked. Express your answer per 100,000 and to the nearest tenth.

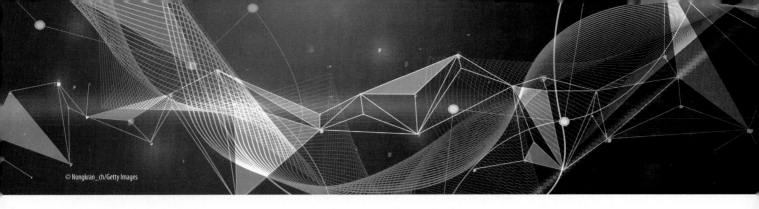

CHAPTER 5

Statistical Inference in Epidemiology

Inferential statistics involves the mathematics of how we generalize or draw conclusions from information obtained from a sample to a population. It is tied to hypothesis testing, where hypothesis testing is about making statements about population values, not sample values. However, we use sample information to evaluate the hypotheses.

The epidemiologic research process begins with a statement about a health problem. The problem is a consequence or an end result. Questions then arise as to whether the problem is real and, if so, why and how it came to exist. Hypothesis testing is useful for quantitatively assessing these questions.

The purpose of this chapter is to present the steps of hypothesis testing, the z-, t-, and chi-square distributions for evaluating hypotheses, and steps for determining appropriate sample size.

▶ Hypothesis Testing

Hypotheses are based on learned and observed evidence from which theories or predictions are made. The process of hypothesis testing begins by formulating the **null hypothesis**, which is some postulated belief about the population; it is what is currently believed, or the status quo. It is a formal basis for a statistical test. The **alternative (or research) hypothesis** gives the opposing conjecture to that of the null hypothesis. The goal is usually to support this hypothesis as being true.

To evaluate whether there is sufficient evidence to support the research hypothesis, we follow six steps:

1. Formulate a statement about the population parameter, called the "null hypothesis" (H_0).
2. Formulate a statement that contradicts the null hypothesis, called the "alternative" or "research hypothesis" (H_a).
3. Select the level of significance for the statistical test that will be used to evaluate the hypotheses. Also, specify the sample size for the study.

4. Select the appropriate test statistic and identify the degrees of freedom and the critical value.
5. Collect the data, estimate the unknown parameter, and calculate the test statistic.
6. Reject or fail to reject the null hypothesis.

A **standardized test statistic** is used to determine whether there is sufficient evidence from a sample to reject the null hypothesis. The test statistic compares results from a sample with a hypothesized value. The general formula for a standardized test statistic is

$$\frac{\text{Statistic} - \text{Parameter}}{\text{Standard deviation or Standard error}}$$

Common standardized test statistics are the *z*-score and the *t*-score.

▶ *z*-Distribution

The *z*-score tells us how many standard deviations an element is from the mean, and it is expressed as follows:

$$z = \frac{x - \mu_0}{\sigma} \quad \text{(Single value)}$$

z is the *z*-score, *x* is the value of the element, μ_0 is the hypothesized population mean, and σ is the population standard deviation.

By way of interpretation, a *z*-score less than 0 is an element less than the mean, a *z*-score greater than zero is an element greater than the mean, and a *z*-score equal to zero is an element equal to 0 (**FIGURE 5.1**). If the *z*-score equals 1, then the element is one standard deviation above the mean, and so on. For the standard normal distribution, 68.27% of the elements have a *z*-score within one standard deviation of the mean, 95.45% of the elements have a *z*-score within two standard deviations of the mean, and 99.73% of the elements have a *z*-score within three standard deviations of the mean.

We are often interested in how the mean of a sample compares with the hypothesized mean in a population. In this case, the *z*-score is expressed as follows:

$$z = \frac{\bar{x} - \mu_0}{\sigma / \sqrt{n}} \quad \text{(Mean value)}$$

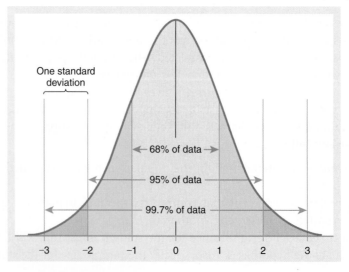

FIGURE 5.1 Distribution of *z*-scores

Here $\bar{x}$ is the sample mean, μ_0 is the population mean under the null hypothesis, σ is the standard deviation of the population, n is the sample size, and $\sigma / \sqrt{n}$ is the standard error. The distribution of z-scores is called the "standard normal distribution." It is a bell-shaped curve with mean 0 and standard deviation 1. It shows the percentage of the population that is between 0 and z, less than z, and greater than z. For example, suppose a sample of 100 adults is taken from a population, and mean body mass index is 27. If the population mean body mass index is 25 and the standard deviation is 15, then

$$z = \frac{27 - 25}{15 / \sqrt{100}} = 1.33$$

The standard normal distribution table shows the area under the curve that corresponds between the mean and the value of the z-score (**TABLE 5.1**). The z-score is measured along the left column and top row of the table. The corresponding area under the curve lies in the body of the table. While the total area under the curve is equal to 1 (because the standard normal distribution is symmetric), the table shows only the upper-right half of the distribution. Thus, the values in the body of the table are the areas between the mean and the value of z.

TABLE 5.1 Standard Normal Distribution Table

z	0	0.01	0.02	0.03	0.04	0.05	0.06	0.07	0.08	0.09
0	0	0.004	0.008	0.012	0.016	0.0199	0.0239	0.0279	0.0319	0.0359
0.1	0.0398	0.0438	0.0478	0.0517	0.0557	0.0596	0.0636	0.0675	0.0714	0.0753
0.2	0.0793	0.0832	0.0871	0.091	0.0948	0.0987	0.1026	0.1064	0.1103	0.1141
0.3	0.1179	0.1217	0.1255	0.1293	0.1331	0.1368	0.1406	0.1443	0.148	0.1517
0.4	0.1554	0.1591	0.1628	0.1664	0.17	0.1736	0.1772	0.1808	0.1844	0.1879
0.5	0.1915	0.195	0.1985	0.2019	0.2054	0.2088	0.2123	0.2157	0.219	0.2224
0.6	0.2257	0.2291	0.2324	0.2357	0.2389	0.2422	0.2454	0.2486	0.2517	0.2549
0.7	0.258	0.2611	0.2642	0.2673	0.2704	0.2734	0.2764	0.2794	0.2823	0.2852
0.8	0.2881	0.291	0.2939	0.2967	0.2995	0.3023	0.3051	0.3078	0.3106	0.3133
0.9	0.3159	0.3186	0.3212	0.3238	0.3264	0.3289	0.3315	0.3304	0.3365	0.3389
1	0.3413	0.3438	0.3461	0.3485	0.3508	0.3531	0.3554	0.3577	0.3599	0.3621
1.1	0.3643	0.3665	0.3686	0.3708	0.3729	0.3749	0.377	0.379	0.381	0.383
1.2	0.3849	0.3869	0.3888	0.3907	0.3925	0.3944	0.3962	0.398	0.3997	0.4015
1.3	0.4032	0.4049	0.4066	0.4082	0.4099	0.4115	0.4131	0.4147	0.4162	0.4177

(continues)

TABLE 5.1 Standard Normal Distribution Table									*(continued)*
z	0	0.01	0.02	0.03	0.04	0.05	0.06	0.07	0.08	0.09
1.4	0.4192	0.4207	0.4222	0.4236	0.4251	0.4265	0.4279	0.4292	0.4306	0.4319
1.5	0.4332	0.4345	0.4357	0.437	0.4382	0.4394	0.4406	0.4418	0.4429	0.4441
1.6	0.4452	0.4463	0.4474	0.4484	0.4495	0.4505	0.4515	0.4525	0.4535	0.4545
1.7	0.4554	0.4564	0.4573	0.4582	0.4591	0.4599	0.4608	0.4616	0.4625	0.4633
1.8	0.4641	0.4649	0.4656	0.4664	0.4671	0.4678	0.4686	0.4693	0.4699	0.4706
1.9	0.4713	0.4719	0.4726	0.4732	0.4738	0.4744	0.475	0.4756	0.4761	0.4767
2	0.4772	0.4778	0.4783	0.4788	0.4793	0.4798	0.4803	0.4808	0.4812	0.4817
2.1	0.4821	0.4826	0.483	0.4834	0.4838	0.4842	0.4846	0.485	0.4854	0.4857
2.2	0.4861	0.4864	0.4868	0.4871	0.4875	0.4878	0.4881	0.4884	0.4887	0.489
2.3	0.4893	0.4896	0.4898	0.4901	0.4904	0.4906	0.4909	0.4911	0.4913	0.4916
2.4	0.4918	0.492	0.4922	0.4925	0.4927	0.4929	0.4931	0.4932	0.4934	0.4936
2.5	0.4938	0.494	0.4941	0.4943	0.4945	0.4946	0.4948	0.4949	0.4951	0.4952
2.6	0.4953	0.4955	0.4956	0.4957	0.4959	0.496	0.4961	0.4962	0.4963	0.4964
2.7	0.4965	0.4966	0.4967	0.4968	0.4969	0.497	0.4971	0.4972	0.4973	0.4974
2.8	0.4974	0.4975	0.4976	0.4977	0.4977	0.4978	0.4979	0.4979	0.498	0.4981
2.9	0.4981	0.4982	0.4982	0.4983	0.4984	0.4984	0.4985	0.4985	0.4986	0.4986
3	0.4987	0.4987	0.4987	0.4988	0.4988	0.4989	0.4989	0.4989	0.499	0.499
3.1	0.499	0.4991	0.4991	0.4991	0.4992	0.4992	0.4992	0.4992	0.4993	0.4993
3.2	0.4993	0.4993	0.4994	0.4994	0.4994	0.4994	0.4994	0.4995	0.4995	0.4995
3.3	0.4995	0.4995	0.4995	0.4996	0.4996	0.4996	0.4996	0.4996	0.4996	0.4997
3.4	0.4997	0.4997	0.4997	0.4997	0.4997	0.4997	0.4997	0.4997	0.4997	0.4998
3.5	0.4998	0.4998	0.4998	0.4998	0.4998	0.4998	0.4998	0.4998	0.4998	0.4998
3.6	0.4998	0.4998	0.4999	0.4999	0.4999	0.4999	0.4999	0.4999	0.4999	0.4999
3.7	0.4999	0.4999	0.4999	0.4999	0.4999	0.4999	0.4999	0.4999	0.4999	0.4999
3.8	0.4999	0.4999	0.4999	0.4999	0.4999	0.4999	0.4999	0.4999	0.4999	0.4999

▶ *t*-Distribution

The second common standardized test statistic is the *t*-score for the mean value of a single population:

$$t = \frac{\bar{x} - \mu_0}{s / \sqrt{n}}$$

The *t*-score for comparing the mean between two independent populations is

$$t = \frac{\bar{x}_1 - \bar{x}_2 - (\mu_1 - \mu_2)}{\sqrt{(s_1^2 / n_1) + (s_2^2 / n_2)}}$$

Both the *z*-score and the *t*-score allow us to compare a statistic to a "normal population." The *t*-score formula looks similar to the *z*-score, but with the *t*-score, we do not know the standard deviation of the population. Because of this, we use *s*, the standard deviation of the sample. In general, we use the *t*-score if the sample size is under 30 and the standard deviation is unknown. The *t*-distribution is flatter and the tails are fatter than the standard normal distribution. As the sample size (or degrees of freedom) increases, the *t*-distribution approaches the *z*-distribution (**FIGURE 5.2**). Percentiles of the *t*-distribution are shown in the following table (**TABLE 5.2**).

Degrees of freedom are the number of independent pieces of information used to obtain an estimate; they are the number of independent observations in a sample minus the number of parameters that are estimated from the sample. For the *t*-statistic, the degrees of freedom are *n* − 1.

The **critical value** is a number from the *t*-distribution that we compare with the value obtained from a test statistic to determine whether or not to reject the null hypothesis. We obtain it from the *t*-distribution table. For example, the critical value for 25 degrees of freedom and a selected level of significance of 0.05 is 1.708 for a one-sided test and 2.06 for a two-sided test. As the sample size increases, corresponding values approach 1.645 and 1.96, respectively. A **one-sided test** is used if the alternative hypothesis is assumed to be greater or less than a specified value. A **two-tailed test** is used if the alternative hypothesis is assumed to equal something. If the calculated test statistic exceeds the critical value, we reject H_0. For example, the mean body mass index for a specific adult population is 25.19. A sample of 26 people is chosen, with mean

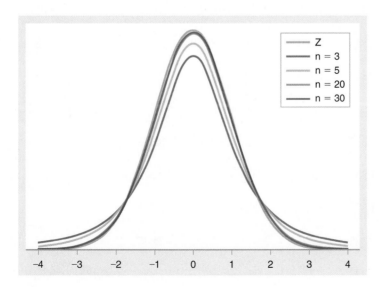

FIGURE 5.2 Distribution of *t*-scores

TABLE 5.2 Percentiles of the *t*-Distribution

One-Sided	75%	80%	85%	90%	95%	97.50%	99%	99.50%	99.75%	99.90%	99.95%
Two-Sided	50%	60%	70%	80%	90%	95%	98%	99%	99.50%	99.80%	99.90%
Degrees of Freedom											
1	1	1.376	1.963	3.078	6.314	12.71	31.82	63.66	127.3	318.3	636.6
2	0.816	1.061	1.386	1.886	2.92	4.303	6.965	9.925	14.09	22.33	31.6
3	0.765	0.978	1.25	1.638	2.353	3.182	4.541	5.841	7.453	10.21	12.92
4	0.741	0.941	1.19	1.533	2.132	2.776	3.747	4.604	5.598	7.173	8.61
5	0.727	0.92	1.156	1.476	2.015	2.571	3.365	4.032	4.773	5.893	6.869
6	0.718	0.906	1.134	1.44	1.943	2.447	3.143	3.707	4.317	5.208	5.959
7	0.711	0.896	1.119	1.415	1.895	2.365	2.998	3.499	4.029	4.785	5.408
8	0.706	0.889	1.108	1.397	1.86	2.306	2.896	3.355	3.833	4.501	5.041
9	0.703	0.883	1.1	1.383	1.833	2.262	2.821	3.25	3.69	4.297	4.781
10	0.7	0.879	1.093	1.372	1.812	2.228	2.764	3.169	3.581	4.144	4.587
11	0.697	0.876	1.088	1.363	1.796	2.201	2.718	3.106	3.497	4.025	4.437
12	0.695	0.873	1.083	1.356	1.782	2.179	2.681	3.055	3.428	3.93	4.318
13	0.694	0.87	1.079	1.35	1.771	2.16	2.65	3.012	3.372	3.852	4.221
14	0.692	0.868	1.076	1.345	1.761	2.145	2.624	2.977	3.326	3.787	4.14
15	0.691	0.866	1.074	1.341	1.753	2.131	2.602	2.947	3.286	3.733	4.073
16	0.69	0.865	1.071	1.337	1.746	2.12	2.583	2.921	3.252	3.686	4.015
17	0.689	0.863	1.069	1.333	1.74	2.11	2.567	2.898	3.222	3.646	3.965
18	0.688	0.862	1.067	1.33	1.734	2.101	2.552	2.878	3.197	3.61	3.922
19	0.688	0.861	1.066	1.328	1.729	2.093	2.539	2.861	3.174	3.579	3.883
20	0.687	0.86	1.064	1.325	1.725	2.086	2.528	2.845	3.153	3.552	3.85
21	0.686	0.859	1.063	1.323	1.721	2.08	2.518	2.831	3.135	3.527	3.819

22	0.686	0.858	1.061	1.321	1.717	2.074	2.508	2.819	3.119	3.505	3.792
23	0.685	0.858	1.06	1.319	1.714	2.069	2.5	2.807	3.104	3.485	3.767
24	0.685	0.857	1.059	1.318	1.711	2.064	2.492	2.797	3.091	3.467	3.745
25	0.684	0.856	1.058	1.316	1.708	2.06	2.485	2.787	3.078	3.45	3.725
26	0.684	0.856	1.058	1.315	1.706	2.056	2.479	2.779	3.067	3.435	3.707
27	0.684	0.855	1.057	1.314	1.703	2.052	2.473	2.771	3.057	3.421	3.69
28	0.683	0.855	1.056	1.313	1.701	2.048	2.467	2.763	3.047	3.408	3.674
29	0.683	0.854	1.055	1.311	1.699	2.045	2.462	2.756	3.038	3.396	3.659
30	0.683	0.854	1.055	1.31	1.697	2.042	2.457	2.75	3.03	3.385	3.646
40	0.681	0.851	1.05	1.303	1.684	2.021	2.423	2.704	2.971	3.307	3.551
50	0.679	0.849	1.047	1.299	1.676	2.009	2.403	2.678	2.937	3.261	3.496
60	0.679	0.848	1.045	1.296	1.671	2	2.39	2.66	2.915	3.232	3.46
80	0.678	0.846	1.043	1.292	1.664	1.99	2.374	2.639	2.887	3.195	3.416
100	0.677	0.845	1.042	1.29	1.66	1.984	2.364	2.626	2.871	3.174	3.39
120	0.677	0.845	1.041	1.289	1.658	1.98	2.358	2.617	2.86	3.16	3.373
∞	0.674	0.842	1.036	1.282	1.645	1.96	2.326	2.576			

27.96 and standard deviation 8.11. We do not know the population standard deviation. What is the standardized test statistic?

$$t = \frac{27.96 - 25.19}{8.11 / \sqrt{26}} = 1.708$$

Now, what about the level of significance? This is a value that is selected by the investigator. It represents the maximum probability we are willing to accept for making a Type I error. There is always the possibility of making a Type I error when using a sample to make inferences (**TABLE 5.3**). The probability of a Type I error is denoted by the Greek letter alpha (α), which is called the **level of significance**. It is typically set at 0.05, as determined by the investigator. Another type of error in hypothesis testing is a Type II error (Table 5.3). The probability of committing a Type II error is denoted by the Greek letter beta (β). It is typically set at 0.20, as determined by the investigator. A related term is the **level of confidence**, which applies when the researcher says that the hypotheses will be accepted only if we can have $(1 - \alpha) \times 100$ confidence that the result actually represents the truth. Although we would prefer α and β to be near 0, this is often not possible. Because the investigator is interested in accepting H_a (rejecting H_0), we are most interested in α being small.

TABLE 5.3 Possible Decisions and Consequences for a Test of Hypothesis

	True State of the Population	
Possible Decisions	H_0 **Is True**	H_a **Is True**
Reject H_0 (accept H_a)	Type I error	Correct decision
Accept H_0	Correct decision	Type II error

In order to reject H_0, the p-value must be lower than the selected α. The p-value is obtained as follows:

1. Calculate the test statistic.
2. Identify its location in an appropriate probability distribution table.
3. Identify the corresponding p-value in the table.

The t-statistic is the appropriate test statistic for evaluating the hypothesized mean value in a single group, assuming the normal distribution.

Hypotheses and test statistics corresponding to various research questions and types of data are presented in **TABLE 5.4**. The hypotheses are limited to one or two group comparisons. When means are compared between three or more groups, a method called **analysis of variance (ANOVA)** is useful, given that certain assumptions are satisfied. When proportions are compared between three or more groups, the χ^2 (chi-squared, pronounced "kaɪsˈkwer") test is used.

▶ χ^2-Distribution

The χ^2-**distribution** is a continuous distribution derived from a sampling distribution of a sum of squares of independent standard normal variables. The distribution is skewed right with only nonnegative values of the variables possible (**FIGURE 5.3**). In the figure, P represents the probability of exceeding the critical value. The shape of the distribution depends on degrees of freedom. The χ^2-distribution is used in epidemiology for estimating selected types of confidence intervals and evaluating hypotheses involving nominal scared data. The χ^2-distribution is shown in **TABLE 5.5**.

▶ Sample Size

You noticed in the previous exercises that sample size is stated in the steps of hypothesis testing. Having an appropriate sample size is critical to the success of any research study. If the sample size is too small, then there may be insufficient information to obtain a correct conclusion. If the sample size is too large, then resources and time are wasted. There are a number of approaches for determining sample size, depending on the type of data employed.

Estimating the sample size for an analytic study requires that we formulate our hypotheses, select a statistical test and identify whether it is a one- or two-sided test, choose the effect size and variability, and specify the values of α and β (**TABLE 5.6**). The effect size and variability can sometimes be estimated from previous studies or consultation with experts. It may also be necessary to obtain

TABLE 5.4 Selected Research Questions, Assumptions, Hypothesis Formulations, and Test Statistics

Research Question …	Data	Assumptions	Possible Forms of the Hypotheses	Test Statistics	Degrees of Freedom
about the mean in one group	Discrete or continuous	Normal population with the variance σ^2 unknown; t-distribution	$H_0 : \mu \geq \mu_0 \quad H_a : \mu < \mu_0$ $H_0 : \mu \leq \mu_0 \quad H_a : \mu > \mu_0$ $H_0 : \mu = \mu_0 \quad H_a : \mu \neq \mu_0$	$t = \dfrac{\bar{x} - \mu_0}{s / \sqrt{n}}$ $s = \sqrt{\dfrac{\sum (x - \bar{x})^2}{n - 1}}$	$n - 1$
about the mean of change scores when the same group is measured twice	Discrete or continuous	Difference score is normally distributed with the variance σ^2 unknown; t-distribution	$H_0 : \delta \geq \delta_0 \quad H_a : \delta < \delta_0$ $H_0 : \delta \leq \delta_0 \quad H_a : \delta > \delta_0$ $H_0 : \delta = \delta_0 \quad H_a : \delta \neq \delta_0$	$t = \dfrac{\bar{d} - \delta_0}{s_d / \sqrt{n}}$ $s_d = \sqrt{\dfrac{\sum (d - \bar{d})^2}{n - 1}}$	$n - 1$
about the proportion in one group	Nominal	The sample size n is at least 30; z-distribution	$H_0 : \pi \geq \pi_0 \quad H_a : \pi < \pi_0$ $H_0 : \pi \leq \pi_0 \quad H_a : \pi > \pi_0$ $H_0 : \pi = \pi_0 \quad H_a : \pi \neq \pi_0$	$z = \dfrac{f - \pi_0}{\sqrt{\pi_0 (1 - \pi_0) / n}}$ f is x/n, the fraction of successes in the sample.	
about the change in proportions when the same group is measured twice	Nominal	The characteristic of interest is measured as a binary scale with r "successes," changed over time; χ^2-distribution	$H_0 : \pi_2 \geq \pi_1 \quad H_a : \pi_2 < \pi_1$ $H_0 : \pi_2 \leq \pi_1 \quad H_a : \pi_2 > \pi_1$ $H_0 : \pi_2 = \pi_1 \quad H_a : \pi_2 \neq \pi_1$	McNemar $\chi^2 = \dfrac{(|b - c|)^2}{b + c}$	$(r - 1)(c - 1)$ r — rows c — columns

(continues)

TABLE 5.4 Selected Research Questions, Assumptions, Hypothesis Formulations, and Test Statistics *(continued)*

Research Question ...	Data	Assumptions	Possible Forms of the Hypotheses	Test Statistics	Degrees of Freedom
about agreement between two observers	Nominal	Cohen's kappa	Interpretation: $k = 0$ no agreement, $k < .4$ indicates poor agreement, $0.4 \leq k < 0.7$ indicates moderate agreement, $0.7 \leq k < 1$ indicates excellent agreement, and $k = 1$ indicates perfect agreement.	$K = \dfrac{2(ad - bc)}{p_1 q_2 + p_2 q_1}$	
about means in two separate groups	Discrete or continuous	The samples are independent random samples. The populations are both normally distributed—this is of less concern when the sample size is at least 30. The population variances (or equivalently, the standard deviations) for both groups are equal.	$H_0 : \mu_1 \geq \mu_2 \quad H_a : \mu_1 < \mu_2$ $H_0 : \mu_1 \leq \mu_2 \quad H_a : \mu_1 > \mu_2$ $H_0 : \mu_1 = \mu_2 \quad H_a : \mu_1 \neq \mu_2$	$t = \dfrac{(\bar{x}_1 - \bar{x}_2) - 0}{s_p \sqrt{(1/n_1) + (1/n_2)}}$ $s_P = \sqrt{\dfrac{(n_1 - 1)s_1^2 + (n_2 - 1)s_2^2}{n_1 + n_2 - 2}}$	$n_1 + n_2 - 2$
about proportions in two independent groups	Nominal	χ^2-distribution	$H_0 : \pi_1 \geq \pi_2 \quad H_a : \pi_1 < \pi_2$ $H_0 : \pi_1 \leq \pi_2 \quad H_a : \pi_1 > \pi_2$ $H_0 : \pi_1 = \pi_2 \quad H_a : \pi_1 \neq \pi_2$	$\chi^2 = \dfrac{(|ad - bc| - n/2)^2 \, n}{(a + b)(c + d)(a + c)(b + d)}$	$(r - 1)(c - 1)$

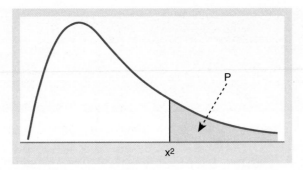

FIGURE 5.3 χ^2-distribution

TABLE 5.5 χ^2-Distribution Table										
	Probability of Exceeding the Critical Value									
df	0.995	0.99	0.975	0.95	0.9	0.1	0.05	0.025	0.01	0.005
1	—	—	0.001	0.004	0.016	2.706	3.841	5.024	6.635	7.879
2	0.01	0.02	0.051	0.103	0.211	4.605	5.991	7.378	9.21	10.597
3	0.072	0.115	0.216	0.352	0.584	6.251	7.815	9.348	11.345	12.838
4	0.207	0.297	0.484	0.711	1.064	7.779	9.488	11.143	13.277	14.86
5	0.412	0.554	0.831	1.145	1.61	9.236	11.07	12.833	15.086	16.75
6	0.676	0.872	1.237	1.635	2.204	10.645	12.592	14.449	16.812	18.548
7	0.989	1.239	1.69	2.167	2.833	12.017	14.067	16.013	18.475	20.278
8	1.344	1.646	2.18	2.733	3.49	13.362	15.507	17.535	20.09	21.955
9	1.735	2.088	2.7	3.325	4.168	14.684	16.919	19.023	21.666	23.589
10	2.156	2.558	3.247	3.94	4.865	15.987	18.307	20.483	23.209	25.188
11	2.603	3.053	3.816	4.575	5.578	17.275	19.675	21.92	24.725	26.757
12	3.074	3.571	4.404	5.226	6.304	18.549	21.026	23.337	26.217	28.3
13	3.565	4.107	5.009	5.892	7.042	19.812	22.362	24.736	27.688	29.819
14	4.075	4.66	5.629	6.571	7.79	21.064	23.685	26.119	29.141	31.319
15	4.601	5.229	6.262	7.261	8.547	22.307	24.996	27.488	30.578	32.801
16	5.142	5.812	6.908	7.962	9.312	23.542	26.296	28.845	32	34.267
17	5.697	6.408	7.564	8.672	10.085	24.769	27.587	30.191	33.409	35.718

(continues)

TABLE 5.5 χ^2-Distribution Table *(continued)*

	Probability of Exceeding the Critical Value									
df	0.995	0.99	0.975	0.95	0.9	0.1	0.05	0.025	0.01	0.005
18	6.265	7.015	8.231	9.39	10.865	25.989	28.869	31.526	34.805	37.156
19	6.844	7.633	8.907	10.117	11.651	27.204	30.144	32.852	36.191	38.582
20	7.434	8.26	9.591	10.851	12.443	28.412	31.41	34.17	37.566	39.997
21	8.034	8.897	10.283	11.591	13.24	29.615	32.671	35.479	38.932	41.401
22	8.643	9.542	10.982	12.338	14.041	30.813	33.924	36.781	40.289	42.796
23	9.26	10.196	11.689	13.091	14.848	32.007	35.172	38.076	41.638	44.181
24	9.886	10.856	12.401	13.848	15.659	33.196	36.415	39.364	42.98	45.559
25	10.52	11.524	13.12	14.611	16.473	34.382	37.652	40.646	44.314	46.928
26	11.16	12.198	13.844	15.379	17.292	35.563	38.885	41.923	45.642	48.29
27	11.808	12.879	14.573	16.151	18.114	36.741	40.113	43.195	46.963	49.645
28	12.461	13.565	15.308	16.928	18.939	37.916	41.337	44.461	48.278	50.993
29	13.121	14.256	16.047	17.708	19.768	39.087	42.557	45.722	49.588	52.336
30	13.787	14.953	16.791	18.493	20.599	40.256	43.773	46.979	50.892	53.672
40	20.707	22.164	24.433	26.509	29.051	51.805	55.758	59.342	63.691	66.766
50	27.991	29.707	32.357	34.764	37.689	63.167	67.505	71.42	76.154	79.49
60	35.534	37.485	40.482	43.188	46.459	74.397	79.082	83.298	88.379	91.952
70	43.275	45.442	48.758	51.739	55.329	85.527	90.531	95.023	100.425	104.215
80	51.172	53.54	57.153	60.391	64.278	96.578	101.879	106.629	112.329	116.321
90	59.196	61.754	65.647	69.126	73.291	107.565	113.145	118.136	124.116	128.299
100	67.328	70.065	74.222	77.929	82.358	118.498	124.342	129.561	135.807	140.169

these estimates using a small pilot study. The effect size may also be selected according to what is clinically meaningful. The specific steps of sample size calculation are:

1. Formulate the null hypothesis.
2. Formulate the alternative hypothesis.
3. Indicate the anticipated effect size.

4. Indicate the measure of variability.
5. Specify the values of α and β.
6. Calculate the sample size using the appropriate formula.

For descriptive epidemiologic studies, hypothesis testing and power are not relevant. Instead, estimating the population parameter is the goal. A descriptive statistic is commonly reported with a confidence interval, which is a range of values around the sample mean or proportion. The confidence interval is a measure of precision of the sample estimate. The sample size equation for estimating a mean is

$$n = \frac{4 \times z_{\alpha/2}^2 s^2}{\text{Width}^2}$$

In particular, use this equation if you are interested in the required sample size for estimating the mean of a continuous variable within $\pm$? points, with ? % confidence.

The sample size equation for estimating a proportion is

$$n = \frac{4 \times z_{\alpha/2}^2 \pi(1 - \pi)}{\text{Width}^2}$$

Specifically, use this equation if you are interested in the required sample size for estimating a proportion with a ? % confidence interval within ± 0.05. The width here is 0.10 and the margin of error is 0.05.

TABLE 5.6 Equations for Estimating Sample Size for Selected Situations

Equation for estimating the sample size for one mean	$n = \left[\dfrac{(z_{\alpha/2} - z_{\beta})\sigma}{\mu_1 - \mu_0} \right]^2$
Equation for estimating the sample size for one proportion	$n = \left[\dfrac{z_{\alpha/2}\sqrt{\pi_0(1 - \pi_0)} - z_{\beta}\sqrt{\pi_1(1 - \pi_1)}}{\pi_1 - \pi_0} \right]^2$
Equation for estimating the sample size for two means	$n = 2\left[\dfrac{(z_{\alpha/2} - z_{\beta})\sigma}{\mu_1 - \mu_0} \right]^2$ n = total number of participants required per group
Equation for estimating the sample size for two proportions	Total sample size required: $n = \left[\dfrac{z_{\alpha/2}\sqrt{4\pi(1 - \pi)} - z_{\beta}\sqrt{2\pi_1(1 - \pi_1) + 2\pi_2(1 - \pi_2)}}{\pi_1 - \pi_2} \right]^2$ The symbol $\pi = (\pi_1 + \pi_2)/2$, π_1 is the proportion in one group, and π_2 is the proportion in the other group. Required sample size per group: $n = \left[\dfrac{z_{\alpha/2}\sqrt{2\pi(1 - \pi)} - z_{\beta}\sqrt{\pi_1(1 - \pi_1) + \pi_2(1 - \pi_2)}}{\pi_1 - \pi_2} \right]^2$

Summary

1. Statistical inference is a conclusion made about a population based on a sample from that population.
2. Hypothesis testing involves statements about population values, but we use sample information to evaluate the hypotheses.
3. The null hypothesis is a postulated belief about the population. The alternative (or research) hypothesis gives the opposing conjecture to that of the null hypothesis.
4. A standardized test statistic is used to determine whether there is sufficient evidence from a sample to reject the null hypothesis. Two common standardized test statistics are the t-score and the z-score. The distribution of z-scores is called the "standard normal distribution." It is a bell-shaped curve with mean 0 and standard deviation 1. The distribution of t-scores looks similar to the distribution of z-scores, but the t-distribution is flatter, with thicker tails.
5. Degrees of freedom are the number of independent pieces of information used to obtain an estimate; they are the number of independent observations in a sample minus the number of parameters that are estimated from the sample.
6. The critical value is a number on the test distribution that we compare to the value obtained from a test statistic to determine whether or not to reject the null hypothesis. The probability of a Type I error is denoted by the Greek letter alpha (α), which is called the "level of significance." The level of confidence is $(1 - \alpha) \times 100$.
7. The specific steps of sample size calculation for an analytic study are: (a) formulate the null hypothesis; (b) formulate the alternative hypothesis; (c) indicate the anticipated effect size; (d) indicate the measure of variability; (e) specify the values of α and β; and (f) calculate the sample size using the appropriate formula.
8. Calculating the sample size for a descriptive study where we do not have hypotheses involves (a) estimate the standard deviation for a continuous variable of interest or the proportion with a dichotomous outcome; (b) specify desired precision (width) of the confidence interval; and (c) specify the confidence level.

Computer Application

1. Open the Excel workbook Application 5.1.xlsx. Compute the mean, standard deviation, standard error, and t-statistic.
2. Open the Excel workbook Application 5.2.xlsx. Review how to compute the answers in Practice Problems 9–19. For Practice Problem 11, obtain the exact p-value and a 95% confidence interval. To proceed, select the STATCALC option in Epi Info and then the Population Binomial tab. In the table, enter the values for the numerator, total observations, and expected percentage. The resulting p-value is 0.0158, and the 95% confidence interval is 72–95.
3. To evaluate Practice Problem 12 using Epi Info, select the STATCALC option and then the Pair-Matched Case-Control Study tab. In the table, enter the values. The resulting two-tailed p-value is 0.1967.
4. Open the Excel workbook Application 5.2.xlsx. Select cell C8 and review how to compute the kappa value in Problem 13.

5. To evaluate Practice Problem 14, open Epi Info and select CLASSIC. In this tab, go to the data folder on the left side of the screen and select Read. We want to import data from an Excel workbook. Under Database Type, select Microsoft Excel 2007 Workbook (.xlsx). Then select Browse and identify Application 5.3.xlsx. Under Data Source Explorer, select Sheet1$ and then click OK. In the Output screen will appear:

    Current Data Source: F:\Application 5.3.xlsx *Record Count:* 674
    (Deleted Records Excluded) Date: 7/14/20172:45:18 PM
    In the Program Editor, you will see:

    READ {F:\Application 5.3.xlsx}

    Select Means and then under Means of, select HealthTest. Under Cross-tabulation by Value of, select Group, and under Stratify by, select Time. Then click OK. For Time 1 (baseline), the mean health test score in the intervention group is 15.95 and in the control group it is 14.84. The means are significantly different, with the p-value = 0.0031. At Time 2 (6 weeks) the means are 23.89 and 15.70, respectively. The means are significantly different, with the p-value < 0.0001.

6. For Practice Problem 15, let's evaluate this problem in Epi Info. To evaluate this problem, select the StatCalc option and then 2×2 Tables. Fill in the table. The resulting p-value is 0.0234, the risk ratio is 1.94, and the 95% confidence interval is 1.16–4.36. The corrected chi-square = 5.1357, with $p = 0.0234$.

7. Open the Excel workbook Application 5.4.xlsx and review how to compute sample size for a descriptive study of a continuous variable (worksheet P20) and of a dichotomous variable (worksheet P21). Now open Epi Info 7, STATCALC, POPULATION SURVEY. For Expected Frequency, type 80, and for Acceptable Margin of Error, type 5. The required sample size of 246 appears next to the confidence level of 95%.

8. Calculating the sample size for a descriptive study where we do not have hypotheses involves (a) estimating the standard deviation for a continuous variable of interest or the proportion with a dichotomous outcome; (b) specifying desired precision (width) of the confidence interval; and (c) specifying the confidence level.

Practice Problems

5.1

Refer to Table 5.1 in the text. Find the probability:

Between 0 and 1.33 _____

Less than 1.33 _____

Greater than 1.33 _____

5.2

Refer to Table 5.1 in the text. What is the z-score that corresponds with 0.975? (Note that because only the upper-right half of the distribution is shown in the table, use 0.475.)

5.3

Refer to Table 5.2 in the text. What is the t-score that corresponds with 0.95 and 1,000 degrees of freedom (two-sided)?

_____

97.5 (one-sided)?

_____

5.4

Refer to Table 5.2 in the text. What is the t-score that corresponds with 0.95 and 10 degrees of freedom (two-sided)?

_____

97.5 (one-sided)?

_____

5.5

Refer to Table 5.2 in the text. What is the area under the curve for the t-distribution up to 1.708?

_____

5.6

Refer to Table 5.2 in the text. What is the area under the curve for the t-distribution above 1.708?

_____

5.7

Refer to Table 5.2 in the text. Suppose we calculate a t-statistic of 2.228, where the alternative hypothesis is one-sided and the degrees of freedom are 10. What is the p-value and conclusion about H_0 (i.e., reject or fail to reject)?

p-value_____

Conclusion about H_0_____

5.8

Refer to Table 5.2 in the text. Suppose that it is commonly believed that the mean percentage of the adult population in the United States who have consumed at least one drink of alcohol within the past 30 days is 50. You would like to see if the actual percentage is different than that value. A sample of 10 states is selected with each state's percentage as follows: 51.3, 40.6, 53.1, 52.1, 40.6, 58.2, 58, 55.1, 50.7, and 54. Assume a normal distribution of mean percentage scores. Evaluate this data using the six steps of hypothesis testing.

For Steps 1 and 2, select from the following:

$$H_0 : \mu = 50\%$$

$$H_a : \mu \neq 50\%$$

$$H_0 : \bar{x} = 50\%$$

$$H_a : \bar{x} \neq 50\%$$

$$H_0 : \mu > 50\%$$

$$H_a : \mu < 50\%$$

$$H_0 : \bar{x} \leq 50\%$$

$$H_a : \bar{x} \geq 50\%$$

1. _____

2. _____

3. $\alpha = $ _____ , $n = $ _____

4. t critical value = _____

5. t calculated value = _____

6. Reject H_0 or fail to reject H_0? _____

Is the p-value greater than or less than 0.05?

_____

5.9

Refer to Table 5.2 in the text. Suppose that it is commonly believed that the mean number of refills on a certain prescribed medication is eight, but you think the true number is different than that. Assume the distribution of prescription refills is normally distributed and the sample size is 126. Let $\bar{x} = 9.5$ and $s = 8$. Evaluate this data using the six steps of hypothesis testing.

For Steps 1 and 2, select from the following:

$$H_0 : \mu = 8$$

$$H_a : \mu \neq 8$$

$$H_0 : \bar{x} = 8$$

$$H_a : \bar{x} \neq 8$$

$$H_0 : \mu > 8$$

$$H_a : \mu < 8$$

$$H_0 : \bar{x} \leq 8$$

$$H_a : \bar{x} \geq 8$$

1. _____

2. _____

3. $\alpha =$ _____ , $n =$ _____

4. t critical value = _____

5. t calculated value = _____

6.   Reject H_0 or fail to reject H_0? _____

Is the p-value greater than or less than 0.05?

_____

5.10

Refer to Table 5.2 in the text. In a study evaluating the efficacy of a coronary heart disease prevention program, researchers wanted to identify whether a decrease in body mass index (BMI) occurred among a group of obese patients over a 6-month period. BMI was measured at the beginning of the study and again at 6 months for each of 50 study participants. From our hypothetical sample of data, $\bar{d} = -0.75$ and $s = 3$. Assume the difference scores are approximately normally distributed. Apply the steps of hypothesis testing.

For Steps 1 and 2, select from the following:

$$H_0 : \delta = 0$$

$$H_a : \delta \neq 0$$

$$H_0 : \bar{\delta} = 0$$

$$H_a : \bar{\delta} \neq 0$$

$$H_0 : \delta > 0$$

$$H_a : \delta < 0$$

$$H_0 : \bar{\delta} \leq 0$$

$$H_a : \bar{\delta} \geq 0$$

1. _____

2. _____

3. $\alpha =$ _____ , $n =$ _____

4. t critical value = _____

5. t calculated value = _____

6.   Reject H_0 or fail to reject H_0? _____

Is the p-value greater than or less than 0.05?

_____

5.11

Refer to Table 5.1 in the text. A researcher is trying to recruit participants for a clinical trial. She believes \$25 would be sufficient to encourage at least 0.70 (or 70%) of a target population to participate. Suppose that in a sample of 136 individuals, 84 choose to participate in the study. Apply the steps of hypothesis testing to this data.

For Steps 1 and 2, select from the following:

$$H_0 : \pi = 0.7$$

$$H_a : \pi \neq 0.7$$

$$H_0 : \pi > 0.7$$

$$H_a : \pi < 0.7$$

$$H_0 : \pi \leq 0.7$$

$$H_a : \pi \geq 0.7$$

1. _____

2. _____

3. $\alpha =$ _____ , $n =$ _____

4. z critical value = _____

5. z calculated value = _____

6. Reject H_0 or fail to reject H_0? _____

Is the p-value greater than or less than 0.05?

_____

5.12

Refer to Table 5.5 in the text. A study was conducted to assess whether an intervention could lower the frequency of the feeling of hopelessness among a selected group of college students. A group of 65 students was selected. They were each asked if they had experienced feelings of hopelessness in the prior week. Then, they received a 4-week intervention. At 6 weeks, they were again asked if they had experienced feelings of hopelessness in the prior week. The following data was collected.

Observed Counts			
	6 Weeks		
Baseline	Yes	No	Total
Yes	20	10	30
No	5	30	35
Total	25	40	65

For Steps 1 and 2, select from the following:

$$H_0 : \pi_2 > \pi_1$$

$$H_a : \pi_2 < \pi_1$$

$$H_0 : \pi_2 = \pi_1$$

$$H_a : \pi_2 \neq \pi_1$$

$$H_0 : \pi_2 \geq \pi_1$$

$$H_a : \pi_2 < \pi_1$$

$$H_0 : \pi_2 \neq \pi_1$$

$$H_a : \pi_2 = \pi_1$$

$$H_0 : \pi_2 \neq \pi_1$$

$$H_a : \pi_2 = \pi_1$$

1. _____

2. _____

3. $\alpha =$ _____ , $n =$ _____

4. McNemar critical value = _____

5. McNemar χ^2 calculated value = _____

6. Reject H_0 or fail to reject H_0? _____

Is the p-value greater than or less than 0.05?

_____

5.13

Suppose two voice specialists assessed 100 selected voice patients for a disorder called "spasmodic dysphonia" (SD).

Observed Counts			
	Specialist 2		
Specialist 1	Yes	No	Total
Yes	34	4	30
No	8	54	70
Total	42	58	100

Calculate and interpret Cohen's kappa (K).

_____

5.14

Refer to Table 5.2 in the text. In a study intended to evaluate the effect of a health behavior intervention, 167 adults were randomly assigned to the intervention and 170 adults were assigned to the control group. The mean health knowledge score was 15.95 (SD = 3.54) in the intervention group and 14.84 (SD = 3.26) in the control group. Assume the test scores in both groups are normally distributed. Apply the six steps of hypothesis testing to evaluate whether there is a difference in means.

For Steps 1 and 2, select from the following:

$$H_0 : \mu_1 > \mu_2$$

$$H_a : \mu_1 < \mu_2$$

$$H_0 : \mu_1 = \mu_2$$

$$H_a : \mu_1 \neq \mu_2$$

$$H_0 : \mu_1 \geq \mu_2$$

$$H_a : \mu_1 < \mu_2$$

$$H_0 : \mu_1 \neq \mu_2$$

$$H_a : \mu_1 = \mu_2$$

$$H_0 : \mu_1 \leq \mu_2$$

$$H_a : \mu_1 \leq \mu_2$$

1. _____

2. _____

3. $\alpha =$ _____ , $n =$ _____

4. t critical value = _____

5. t calculated value = _____

6. Reject H_0 or fail to reject H_0? _____

Is the p-value greater than or less than 0.05?

5.15

Refer to Table 5.5 in the text. We are studying whether patients with obstructive sleep apnea (OSA) have a greater chance of having a voice disorder. Suppose that among 125 patients with OSA, 31 have a voice disorder, and that among 125 patients without OSA, 16 have a voice disorder. Apply the steps of hypothesis testing to this data.

For Steps 1 and 2, select from the following:

$$H_0 : \pi_1 > \pi_2$$

$$H_a : \pi_1 < \pi_2$$

$$H_0 : \pi_1 = \pi_2$$

$$H_a : \pi_1 \neq \pi_2$$

$$H_0 : \pi_1 \geq \pi_2$$

$$H_a : \pi_1 < \pi_2$$

$$H_0 : \pi_1 \neq \mu_2$$

$$H_a : \pi_1 = \pi_2$$

$$H_0 : \pi_1 \leq \pi_2$$

$$H_a : \pi_1 \leq \pi_2$$

1. _____

2. _____

3. $\alpha = $ _____ , $n = $ _____

4. χ^2 critical value = _____

5. χ^2 calculated value = _____

6. Reject H_0 or fail to reject H_0? _____

Is the p-value greater than or less than 0.05?

_____

5.16

Refer to Table 5.1 in the text. A study evaluated whether a health intervention could cause a decrease over 6 months in the mean number of refills of a certain prescription medication. Suppose that prior to the study, the investigators wanted to know whether the mean number of prescription refills is different than 8 by either plus or minus 2. Assume a standard deviation of 8. Apply the steps of sample size calculation, with $\alpha = 0.05$ and $\beta = 0.20$.

For Steps 1 and 2, select from the following:

$$H_0 : \bar{x} = 8$$

$$H_a : \bar{x} \neq 8$$

$$H_0 : \mu > 8$$

$$H_a : \mu < 8$$

$$H_0 : \bar{x} \leq 8$$

$$H_a : \bar{x} \geq 8$$

$$H_0 : \mu = 8$$

$$H_a : \mu \neq 8$$

1. _____

2. _____

3. _____ or more

4. Standard deviation = _____

5. α = _____ and β = _____

6. n = _____

5.17

Refer to Table 5.1 in the text. In the past, it was assumed that $25 was a sufficient incentive to encourage at least 0.70 of a target population to participate. However, you suspect the percentage is now lower, no more than 0.50. Apply the steps of hypothesis testing to this data, with $\alpha = 0.05$ and $\beta = 0.20$.

For Steps 1 and 2, select from the following:

$$H_0 : \pi \geq 0.7$$

$$H_a : \pi \geq 0.7$$

$$H_0 : \pi = 0.7$$

$$H_a : \pi \neq 0.7$$

$$H_0 : \pi \geq 0.7$$

$$H_a : \pi \geq 0.7$$

$$H_0 : \pi < 0.7$$

$$H_a : \pi < 0.7$$

$$H_0 : \pi > 0.7$$

$$H_a : \pi > 0.7$$

1. _____

2. _____

3. Assumed truth = _____

4. Standard deviation = _____

5. α = _____ and β = _____

6. n = _____

5.18

Refer to Table 5.1 in the text. Suppose that a new drug has been developed for treating HIV. Researchers want to test whether it is better than an existing treatment at increasing CD4 cell counts. A randomized trial is planned to evaluate the drug. Assume an anticipated effect size of 50, a standard deviation of 100, $\alpha = 0.05$, and $\beta = 0.20$. What is the required sample size per group?

For Steps 1 and 2, select from the following:

$$H_0 : \mu_1 > \mu_2$$

$$H_a : \mu_1 < \mu_2$$

$$H_0 : \mu_1 = \mu_2$$

$$H_a : \mu_1 \neq \mu_2$$

$$H_0 : \mu_1 \geq \mu_2$$

$$H_a : \mu_1 < \mu_2$$

$$H_0 : \mu_1 \neq \mu_2$$

$$H_a : \mu_1 = \mu_2$$

$$H_0 : \mu_1 \leq \mu_2$$

$$H_a : \mu_1 \leq \mu_2$$

1. _____

2. _____

3. Difference in means = _____

4. Standard deviation = _____

5. $\alpha =$ _____ and $\beta =$ _____

6. $n =$ _____

5.19

Refer to Table 5.1 in the text. Previous research suggests that patients with obstructive sleep apnea (OSA) have a greater chance of having a voice disorder. A literature review suggests that the prevalence of a voice disorder in the general adult population is 0.15. From our experience, it is about 0.30 among patients with OSA. Apply the steps of sample size calculation to determine the number of participants required to evaluate whether OSA is associated with an increased risk of a voice disorder.

For Steps 1 and 2, select from the following:

$$H_0 : \pi_1 > \pi_2$$

$$H_a : \pi_1 < \pi_2$$

$$H_0 : \pi_1 = \pi_2$$

$$H_a : \pi_1 \neq \pi_2$$

$$H_0 : \pi_1 \geq \pi_2$$

$$H_a : \pi_1 < \pi_2$$

$$H_0 : \pi_1 \neq \mu_2$$

$$H_a : \pi_1 = \pi_2$$

$$H_0 : \pi_1 \leq \pi_2$$

$$H_a : \pi_1 \leq \pi_2$$

1. _____

2. _____

3. Difference between _____ and _____ percent

4. Does the null hypothesis assume the proportions are <u>equal</u> or <u>not equal</u>?

_____

5. $\alpha =$ _____ and $\beta =$ _____

6. $\pi =$ _____

7. $n =$ _____

5.20

Refer to Table 5.1 in the text. We are interested in requiring a 95% confidence interval for the mean of a continuous variable. In order to estimate the mean of a continuous variable (SD = 10) with a 95% confidence interval no wider than 5, how many participants are required?

_____

5.21

Refer to Table 5.1 in the text. We are interested in determining the required sample size for estimating the sensitivity of a test at an 80% and 95% confidence interval for the test's sensitivity of ±0.05. How many participants are required?

_____

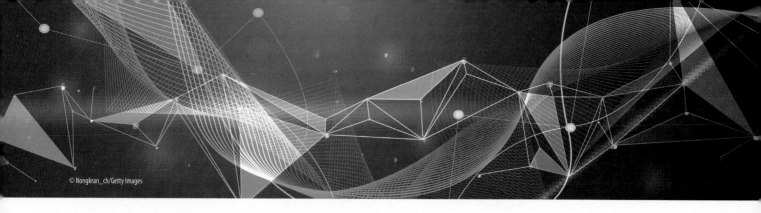

CHAPTER 6

Measures of Association in Epidemiology

There are a number of study designs commonly applied in epidemiology, including the case study, ecologic study, cross-sectional study, case-control study, cohort study, and experimental study. Each of these study designs have strengths and weaknesses and involve specific types of data and measures of association. The purpose of this chapter is to provide a description of each of these study designs and present the types of data and measures of association they employ.

▶ Epidemiologic Study Designs

A study design is a formal approach to scientific and scholarly investigation. It is used to provide direction along the path of systematically collecting, analyzing, and interpreting data. There are both descriptive and analytic study designs in epidemiology. All of the study designs are observational except for the experimental study design, where the level of exposure is assigned and controlled by the researcher.

Study Designs

A list of selected study designs commonly used in epidemiology, along with their strengths and weaknesses, is presented in **TABLE 6.1**. The purpose of the descriptive study design is to describe what is happening. The analytic study design seeks to test hypotheses about associations between variables. The case study is a qualitative description of a problem or situation for an individual or small group. Because a single variable is involved, a measure of association is not relevant. Ecologic and cross-sectional study designs often provide descriptions of things; however, they can also be used to test hypotheses, if the relationship between two or more variables is being evaluated. The ecologic study design reflects aggregate data, wherein there is no specific information available on the individual level. The cross-sectional study design measures variables at

TABLE 6.1 Description of Selected Study Designs with Their Strengths and Weaknesses

	Description	Strengths	Weaknesses
Case study	A snapshot description of a problem or situation for an individual or group; qualitative descriptive research of the facts presented in chronological order.	In-depth description; provides clues to identify a new disease or adverse health effect resulting from an exposure or experience; identifies potential areas of research.	Conclusions limited to the individual, group, and/or context under study; cannot be used to establish a cause–effect relationship.
Ecological	Aggregate data is involved (i.e., no information is available for specific individuals); shows the prevalence of a potential risk factor compared with the rate of an outcome condition.	Takes advantage of preexisting data; relatively quick and inexpensive; can be used to evaluate programs, policies, or regulations implemented at the ecologic level; allows estimation of effects not easily measurable for individuals.	Susceptible to confounding; exposures and disease or injury outcomes are not measured on the same individuals.
Cross-sectional	All of the variables are measured at the same point in time; no distinction is made between potential risk factors and outcomes; an effective way to collect prevalence data.	Control over study population; control over measurements; several associations between variables can be studied at the same time; short time period required; complete data collection; exposure and injury/disease data collected from the same individuals; produces prevalence data.	No data on the time relationship between exposure and injury/disease development; no follow-up; potential bias from low response rate; potential measurement bias; higher proportion of long-term survivors; not feasible with rare exposures or outcomes; does not yield incidence or relative risk.
Case-control	Presence of risk factor(s) for people with a condition is compared with that for people without the condition.	Effective for rare outcomes; compared to a cohort study, requires less time, money, and size; yields the odds ratio (when the outcome condition is rare, a good estimate of the relative risk).	Limited to one outcome condition; does not provide incidence, relative risk, or natural history; less effective than a cohort study at establishing the time sequence of events; potential recall and interviewer bias; potential survival bias; does not yield incidence or prevalence.

Cohort	People are followed over time to describe the incidence or the natural history of a condition; assessment can also be made of risk factors for various conditions.	Establishes time sequence of events; avoids bias in measuring exposure from knowing the outcome; avoids Berkson's bias and prevalence–incidence bias; several outcomes can be assessed; number of outcomes grows over time; allows assessment of incidence and the natural history of disease; yields incidence, relative risk, attributable risk.	Large samples often required; may not be feasible in terms of time and money; not feasible with rare outcomes; limited to one risk factor; potential bias caused by loss of follow-up.
Experimental (or intervention) study	A type of cohort study in which the effects of an assigned intervention on an outcome are evaluated; if conducted in a medical setting to assess a new drug, medical device, or procedure, it is called a "clinical trial"; other types of trials are prophylactic, therapeutic, and community.	The investigators control the exposure levels; sometimes produces a faster and cheaper answer to the research question than observational studies; if individuals or groups can be assigned randomly, then confounding can be controlled; if blinding can be used, then certain biases are minimized.	Only appropriate approach for some research questions; may not be feasible because of ethical barriers or rare outcomes; randomization may not be acceptable; research question may not be suitable for blinding; generalization of the results may be limited because of use of volunteers, eligibility criteria, and loss of follow-up.

a point in time on the individual level. Case-control, cohort, and experimental study designs are generally used to assess hypotheses, although in some cases they are descriptive. The case-control study involves identifying people according to outcome status and then exploring previous exposure status. The cohort study design involves identifying people according to exposure status and then following them over time in order to ascertain outcome status. The experimental (also called "intervention") study is a scientific experiment involving human subjects where an intervention is initiated for therapy evaluation. The key distinction between the descriptive and analytic study design is that the latter is used to test hypotheses, which requires a comparison group.

▶ Measures of Association

A measure of association produces a quantity of the relationship between variables, such as an exposure and disease outcome. The type of measure used depends on the selected design of the study and the type of data employed (**TABLE 6.2**). Not all combinations of exposure and outcome data types are

TABLE 6.2 Measures of Association Used with Types of Exposure and Outcome Data

	Exposure/Outcome			
Study design	Nominal (two levels) / Nominal (two levels)	Nominal (two levels) / Continuous, normally distributed	Continuous, normally distributed / Continuous, normally distributed	Continuous, not normally distributed or ordinal with > two categories / Continuous, not normally distributed or ordinal with > two categories
Ecological	Odds ratio; logistic regression	Comparison of means	Correlation coefficient; linear regression	Spearman rank correlation
Cross-sectional	Prevalence ratio; prevalence difference	Comparison of means	Correlation coefficient; linear regression	Spearman rank correlation
Case-control	Odds ratio; logistic regression			
Cohort / experimental	Risk ratio; risk difference; rate ratio; rate difference; Poisson regression	Comparison of means	Correlation coefficient; linear regression	Spearman rank correlation

TABLE 6.3 2 × 2 Contingency Table Displaying Exposure and Outcome Data

	Case	**Non-Case**
Exposed	a	b
Not exposed	c	d

reflected in the table, but common combinations are listed. The three types of regression models listed are used to estimate slope coefficients, which measure the strength of the association between variables.

To begin, consider the following 2 × 2 contingency table, which is a common way to express the data relationship between two nominal (two-level) scale variables (**TABLE 6.3**). Let a be the number of cases exposed, b be the number of non-cases exposed, c be the number of cases not exposed, and d be the number of non-cases not exposed.

We are often interested in comparing the risk (or rate, or prevalence) between groups. To do this, we can either take the ratio of two risks (or rates, or prevalences) to provide a relative measure of the effect of the exposure, or we can take the difference of two risks (or rates, or prevalences) to provide an absolute measure of the effect of the exposure. Risk (or rate) ratios are measures of association that can be derived from cohort data. Prevalence ratios are derived from cross-sectional data.

▶ Nominal Data

Suppose the data in the table represent exposure and outcome information from a cohort. The risk ratio consists of the incidence rate of the outcome for those exposed divided by the incidence of the outcome for those not exposed.

Let

R_e = the risk or rate of the outcome in the exposed group: $P(\text{Outcome}\,|\,\text{Exposed}) = a/(a + b)$

R_o = the risk or rate of the outcome in the nonexposed group: $P(\text{Outcome}\,|\,\text{Not exposed}) = c/(c + d)$

R = the risk or rate of the outcome in the whole group: $P(\text{Outcome}) = (a + c)/(a + b + c + d)$

The formula is

$$\text{Risk ratio} = \frac{P(\text{Outcome}\,|\,\text{Exposed})}{P(\text{Outcome}\,|\,\text{Not exposed})} = \frac{R_e}{R_o}$$

The 95% confidence interval for a risk ratio is derived as follows:

$$95\%\,\text{CI(RR)} = e^{\ln(\text{Risk ratio}) \pm \left(1.96 \times \sqrt{\frac{b/a}{a+b} + \frac{d/c}{c+d}} \right)}$$

In some cases, we are interested in measuring a rate, where the numerator in the calculation represents new cases for an observation period and the denominator represents the time each person is observed, totaled for all persons (person-time).

	Cases	Non-Cases	Person–Time
Exposed	a	b	PT_e
Not exposed	c	d	PT_o

Let

R_e = the risk or rate of the outcome in the exposed group: $P(\text{Outcome}\,|\,\text{Exposed}) = a/PT_e$

R_o = the risk or rate of the outcome in the nonexposed group: $P(\text{Outcome}\,|\,\text{Not exposed}) = c/PT_o$

R = the risk or rate of the outcome in the whole group: $P(\text{Outcome}) = (a + c)/(PT_e + PT_o)$

The formula is

$$\text{Rate ratio} = \frac{P(\text{Outcome}\,|\,\text{Exposed})}{P(\text{Outcome}\,|\,\text{Not exposed})} = \frac{R_e}{R_o}$$

The 95% confidence interval for a rate ratio is

$$95\%\,\text{CI(RR)} = e^{\ln(\text{Rate ratio}) \pm \left(1.96 \times \sqrt{(1/a) + (1/c)} \right)}$$

The risk (or rate) difference is the difference in the two risks (or rates).

$$RD = P(\text{Outcome}|\text{Exposed}) - P(\text{Outcome}|\text{Not exposed}) = R_e - R_o$$

Two other measures of association are the attributable fraction in the population (also called the "population attributable risk percent") and the attributable fraction in exposed cases (also called the "attributable risk percent").

Attributable Fraction in the Population

$$AF_p = \frac{R - R_o}{R} \times 100$$

This measure reflects the expected proportional reduction in risk that would occur if the exposure were removed from the population. The numerator in the AF_p is the excess of disease in the population attributed to the exposure. For example, $AF_p = 30\%$ means that eliminating the exposure from the population would reduce the number of cases by 30%.

Attributable Fraction in the Exposed Cases

$$AF_e = \frac{R_e - R_o}{R_e} \times 100$$

This measure reflects the expected proportional reduction in cases who were exposed had the exposure not occurred. The numerator in the AF_e is the excess of disease among the exposed group attributed to the exposure. For example, $AF_e = 50\%$ means that among cases who were exposed, 50% of those cases are attributed to their exposure. Both the attributable fraction in the population and the attributable fraction in the exposed cases assumes a causal association between the exposure and outcome variables.

If the data in the table represents the prevalence (all existing cases) of the disease or event at a point in time, then the prevalence for people exposed versus not exposed is calculated in the same way as the risk ratio.

Now suppose the data in the table represents case-control data and, thus, the odds ratio is the appropriate measure of association.

$$\text{Odds ratio} = \frac{P(\text{Exposed}|\text{Outcome}) / P(\text{Not exposed}|\text{Outcome})}{P(\text{Exposed}|\text{No outcome}) / P(\text{Not exposed}|\text{No outcome})}$$
$$= \frac{a/c}{b/d} = \frac{a \times d}{b \times d}$$

The 95% confidence interval for an odds ratio is

$$95\% \text{ CI(OR)} = e^{\ln(\text{Odds ratio}) \pm \left(1.96 \times \sqrt{(1/a) + (1/b) + (1/c) + (1/d)}\right)}$$

The attributable fraction in exposed cases in a case-control study is obtained as:

$$AF_e = \frac{OR - 1}{OR} \times 100$$

The attributable fraction in the population is

$$AF_p = \frac{p_o(OR - 1)}{p_o(OR - 1) + 1} \times 100$$

$$p_o = \frac{c}{c+d}$$

Dependency Ratio

A measure in epidemiology called the **dependency ratio** describes the relationship between those with the potential to be self-supporting and the dependent segments of the population. The formula is

$$\frac{\text{Population} < 15 \text{ and} \geq 65}{\text{Population } 15-64} \times 100$$

▶ Numerical Data

If two numerical (discrete or continuous) variables are obtained, a scatter plot is an appropriate way to display the data. The scatter plot can tell us whether the variables are normally distributed and linearly related. The correlation coefficient and the regression model are standard techniques to measure the association between numerical variables.

In the absence of a linear association, the investigator may choose to apply the correlation measure over a subsection of the data where linearity holds, or use the **Spearman rank correlation coefficient**, which is a measure of association between the ranking of two variables. The **correlation coefficient** measures the strength of the linear association between two variables. It assumes that both variables are normally distributed and that a linear association exists between the variables. The correlation coefficient is a scaled range from −1 (perfect negative association) and +1 (perfect positive association). A 0 value means there is no association between the variables. To calculate the correlation coefficient for a sample, we use the following formula:

$$r = \frac{\sum (x_i - \bar{x})(y_i - \bar{y})}{\sqrt{\sum (x_i - \bar{x})^2 (y_i - \bar{y})^2}}$$

Recall that in a sample, the population parameter ρ (the lowercase Greek letter rho) is estimated by r.

The **coefficient of determination** is a related measure, which is the correlation coefficient squared (denoted as r^2). This measure represents the proportion of the total variation in the outcome variable y that is determined by the exposure variable x. If $r = 1$, then all of the variation in the outcome variable is explained by the exposure variable. However, typically only part of the variation in the outcome variable will be explained by a single variable.

If the population parameter ρ is set to 0 in the null hypothesis, the following mathematical expression involving the correlation coefficient, called the t-ratio, has a t-distribution with $n - 2$ degrees of freedom:

$$t = \frac{r\sqrt{n-2}}{\sqrt{1-r^2}}$$

In the following example, prevalence data from 50 American states was collected. The variable on the vertical axis represents the percentage of the adults aged 50 years and older who had ever had a sigmoidoscopy or colonoscopy (**FIGURE 6.1**). The variable on the horizontal axis represents the percentage of

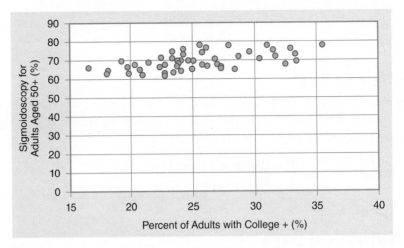

FIGURE 6.1 Colon cancer screening in American states

Data from Centers for Disease Control and Prevention, National Center for Chronic Disease Prevention and Health Promotion, Division of Population Health. BRFSS Prevalence & Trends Data [online]. 2015. [accessed Feb 16, 2017]. URL: https://www.cdc.gov/brfss/brfssprevalence/

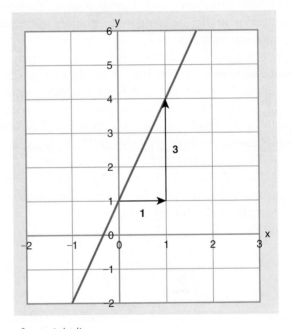

FIGURE 6.2 Slope of a straight line

adults who have had at least some college education. The relationship between these ecologic variables is positive and linear. The estimated correlation coefficient is 0.56, meaning there is a positive association between sigmoidoscopy and education. The coefficient of determination is 0.31, meaning that 31% of the variation in sigmoidoscopy is explained by the education variable.

The slope (gradient) of a straight line in mathematics is the rise over the run. In the following graph (**FIGURE 6.2**), the slope is $3/1 = 3$. In this example, the equation is $y = f(x) = 1 + 3x$. The functional relationship is a perfect relationship. In contrast, a statistical relationship is generally not a perfect one in which each observation falls on the line, but there is a scattering of points about the line. In statistics, we use a technique called "regression" to provide the line that fits best to the data.

Regression analysis plays a central role in epidemiologic research. A primary strength of this technique is that it can be used to estimate the association between variables that are generally not perfectly associated. The method is also useful for assessing associations between variables while controlling for the confounding influence of other variables. A regression model is used to estimate the association between two variables (such as an exposure and outcome), and, unlike the correlation coefficient, produces an estimate that reflects the original data scale. Specifically, this estimate is of the change in the outcome variable (Y) per unit change in the exposure variable (X). This method assumes that (1) for each value of X, Y is normally distributed, , (2) the standard deviation of the outcomes Y do not change over X, (3) the outcomes Y are independent, and (4) a linear relationship exists between X and Y. Data transformations and other methods may be used to respond to violations of these assumptions, which will be covered in future study.

Simple linear regression involves an equation with one explanatory variable. This method fits a linear line to the data that minimizes the squared deviations of each point from the estimated straight line. The equation is

$$Y = \beta_0 + \beta_1 X + \epsilon$$

If y_i is the observed outcome of Y_i for a particular value x_i, and $\hat{y}_i$ is the corresponding predicted value, then

$$e_i = y_i - \hat{y}_i$$

The distance e_i is known as the **residual**. When the regression equation is used to describe the relationship in the sample, it is often written as

$$\hat{y} = b_0 + b_1 x$$

In this equation, b_0 represents the estimated y-intercept of the linear fitted line, and b_1 represents the estimated slope. The slope is a measure of association that indicates how y changes when x changes by one unit. To estimate the intercept and slope, we use the following formulas:

$$b_1 = \frac{\sum (x - \bar{x})(y - \bar{y})}{\sum (x - \bar{x})^2}$$

$$b_0 = \bar{y} - b_1 \bar{x}$$

If the population parameter β_1 is set to 0 in the null hypothesis, the following mathematical expression involving the slope coefficient has a t-distribution with $n - 2$ degrees of freedom:

$$t = \frac{b_1 - 0}{SE_{b_1}}$$

$$SE_{b_1} = \sqrt{\frac{(1/n - 2)\sum (y - \hat{y})^2}{\sum (x - \bar{x})^2}}$$

Note the relationship between the correlation coefficient and the slope coefficient:

$$b_1 = r \frac{\sqrt{\sum (y - \bar{y})^2}}{\sqrt{\sum (x - \bar{x})^2}}$$

$$r = b_1 \frac{\sqrt{\sum (x - \bar{x})^2}}{\sqrt{\sum (y - \bar{y})^2}}$$

The t-statistic for evaluating the slope coefficient in the regression model is expressed as follows:

$$t = \frac{b_1 - \beta_1}{SE_{b_1}}$$

This expression follows the t-distribution with $n - 2$ degrees of freedom under the assumptions of the regression model and is used to test $H_0 : \beta_1 = 0$ against $H_a : \beta_1 \neq 0$.

An extension of the estimated simple linear regression model is the multiple linear regression model:

$$y = b_0 + b_1 x_1 + b_2 x_2 + \cdots + b_k x_k$$

The slope estimate b_1 is interpreted as the change in y mean value per unit change in x_1, adjusted for the other variables in the model. For example, let y = pulse, x_1 = aerobic exercise per week in hours, x_2 = age, and x_3 = body mass index (BMI). Consider the estimated regression line:

$$y = 58 - 1.08x_1 + 0.5x_2 - 0.75x_2$$

The interpretation of b_1 is that for each hour increase in hours exercised, pulse goes down an average of 1.08, after adjusting for age and BMI. Age is a potential confounder of the relationship between exercise and pulse because it is independently related to both. Body mass index is also a potential confounder, for the same reason. You will learn how to estimate multiple regression models in future classes.

If the outcome variable is dichotomous (two levels) rather than numerical, then an alternative regression technique is necessary, called **logistic regression**. Logistic regression is commonly used in epidemiology because many of the outcome measures considered involve nominally scaled data (e.g., ill/not ill, injured/not injured, disabled/not disabled, dead/alive). The slope coefficient is also related to the odd ratio, as will be shown. Let π represent the probability in the population of being a case (such as ill, injured, disabled, or dead) and $1 - \pi$ the probability of not being a case. Then the simple regression model looks like the following:

$$\pi = \beta_0 + \beta_1 X + \epsilon$$

The assumption presented earlier for regression—that Y is normally distributed for each value of X—is violated because π is a probability that ranges from 0 to 1. However, we can modify the outcome variable as follows:

$$\log_e[\text{Odds}] = \ln\left[\frac{\pi}{1 - \pi}\right]$$

This expression is called the "log odds," which is normally distributed and linearly related to the exposure variable X in the following model:

$$\ln\left[\frac{\pi}{1 - \pi}\right] = \beta_0 + \beta_1 X + \epsilon$$

When the logistic regression model is used to describe the relationship in a sample, it is written as

$$\ln\left[\frac{p}{1 - p}\right] = b_0 + b_1 x$$

The slope coefficient b_1 is interpreted as the change in the log odds of the outcome per unit change in x.

Consider b_1 in a logistic model when X is a dichotomous variable that equals 1 if exposed and 0 if not exposed, as follows:

$$\ln(\text{Odds})_e = b_0 + b_1 \times 1$$
$$\ln(\text{Odds})_o = b_0 + b_1 \times 0$$
$$b_1 = \ln(\text{Odds})_e - \ln(\text{Odds})_{ne} = \ln[\text{Odds ratio}]$$
$$\text{Odds ratio} = e^{b_1}$$

e^{b_1} is the odds ratio comparing exposed and not exposed groups.

$$95\% \text{ CI(Odds ratio)} = \exp\left[\ln(\text{Odds ratio}) \pm 1.96\sqrt{\frac{1}{a} + \frac{1}{b} + \frac{1}{c} + \frac{1}{d}}\right]$$

A community-based study of respiratory illness during the first year of life was conducted in South Carolina. As part of this study, a group of children were classified according to family socioeconomic status. The numbers of children in each group who experienced persistent respiratory symptoms are shown as follows:

Socioeconomic Status	Number of Children with Symptoms	Number of Children	Odds Ratio	95% CI
Low	31	79	1.00	—
Middle	29	122	0.61	0.34–1.08
High	27	192	0.36	0.20–0.64

Poisson regression is another important statistical tool frequently used in epidemiology. Poisson regression is appropriate when the dependent events occur infrequently, the events occur independently, and the events occur over some continuous medium such as time or area. The probability of a single event occurring is influenced by the length of the interval. Counts or rates of rare diseases in large populations are well suited for modeling with Poisson regression, such as specific types of cancer.

To describe the meaning of b_1 in a Poisson model when x_1 is a dichotomous variable equal to 1 if exposed and 0 if unexposed,

$$\ln(\text{Rate})_e = b_0 + b_1 \times 1$$
$$\ln(\text{Rate})_{ne} = b_0 + b_1 \times 0$$
$$b_1 = \ln(\text{Rate})_e - \ln(\text{Rate})_{ne} = \ln[\text{Rate ratio}]$$
$$\text{Rate ratio} = e^{b_1}$$

$$95\% \text{ CI(Rate ratio)} = \exp\left[\ln(\text{Rate ratio}) \pm 1.96\sqrt{\frac{1}{a} + \frac{1}{c}}\right]$$

In general, the slope coefficient b_1 is interpreted as the change in the log rates of the outcome per unit change in x. In this example, e^{b_1} is the rate ratio comparing exposed and unexposed groups. If additional variables were included in the models, then the rate ratio $= e^{b_1}$ is adjusted for those variables.

Summary

1. A study design is used to provide direction along the path of systematically collecting, analyzing, and interpreting data. There are both descriptive and analytic study designs in epidemiology. Observational study designs include the case study, ecologic study, cross-sectional study, case-control study, and cohort study. The experimental study design is not an observational study because the exposure level is assigned and controlled by the researcher.

2. The case study is a qualitative description of a problem or situation for an individual or small group; the ecologic study design reflects aggregate data; the cross-sectional study design measures variables at a point in time on the individual level; the case-control study involves identifying people according to outcome status and then exploring previous exposure status; the cohort study design involves identifying people according to exposure status and then following them over time to evaluate outcome status; the experimental (intervention) study is a scientific experiment involving human subjects where treatment is initiated for therapy evaluation.

3. A measure of association produces a quantity of the relationship between variables (such as an exposure and outcome), depending on the study design and data type involved.

4. The risk ratio is a measure of association between an exposure measured on two levels (yes, no) and an outcome measured on two levels (yes, no) in a cohort study. It is the ratio of the risk of the outcome among the exposed group compared with the risk of the outcome in the unexposed group. The risk difference is the risk of the outcome in the exposed group minus the risk of the outcome in the unexposed group.

5. The rate ratio is a measure of association involving the person–time rate of an outcome for people exposed compared with the person–time rate of an outcome for persons not exposed in a cohort study. The rate difference is the rate of the outcome in the exposed group minus the rate of the outcome in the unexposed group.

6. Two other measures that can be obtained from cohort data are the attributable fraction in the population and the attributable fraction in the exposed group. The attributable fraction in the population reflects the expected proportional reduction in risk that would occur if the exposure were removed from the population. The attributable fraction in the exposed group reflects the expected proportional reduction in cases who were exposed had the exposure not occurred.

7. The odds ratio is a measure of the association of the odds of exposure among the cases divided by the odds of the exposure among the non-cases. It is an estimate of the risk ratio, approaching the risk ratio when the outcome is rare.

8. Three types of regression introduced in this chapter include linear regression, logistic regression, and Poisson regression. Linear regression models the relationship between an outcome (or dependent) variable and one or more explanatory (or independent) variables. When there is only one explanatory variable, this model is referred to as "simple linear regression" (compared with multiple linear regression). Logistic

regression models the relationship between an outcome variable and one or more explanatory variables, but the outcome variable has only two possible levels (i.e., it is a dichotomous variable). The exponent of the estimated relationship (slope coefficient) is the odds ratio. Poisson regression assumes that the outcome variable has a Poisson distribution. This is appropriate for studying the counts or rates of rare diseases in large populations.

9. The correlation coefficient is a number between −1 and 1, which represents the strength of the linear association between two numerical variables. If the association is not linear, then Spearman's rank correlation coefficient is a more appropriate measure of association between two numerical variables.

Computer Application

1. Open the Excel workbook Application 6.1.xlsx and review how to compute Practice Problems 1–12.

2. For Practice Problems 1 and 7, open Epi Info and select STATCALC. Then choose TABLES ($2 \times 2 \times N$) and redo the first problem in this chapter, which involved calculating and interpreting the risk ratio for $a = 16$, $b = 8$, $c = 6$, and $d = 20$. For Practice Problem 1, what is the Risk Ratio, 95% confidence interval, corrected chi-square, and p-value? For Problem 7, what is the Odds Ratio, 95% confidence interval, corrected chi-square, and p-value? Is the odds ratio a good estimate of the risk ratio? Why?

3. Open the Excel workbook Application 6.2.xlsx and compute the correlation coefficient and linear regression line for the data in Figure 6.1. Duplicate the graph in Excel. Now open Epi Info and select the VISUAL DASHBOARD and open F:\Application 6.2.xlsx. Under Data Source Explorer, select Question$, and click OK. Click the mouse and select Add Analysis Gadget, Charts, and then Scatter Chart. Enter College as the main variable and Sigmoidoscopy as the outcome variable, and click OK. This will show you a scatter chart of the assocation between our two variables. The linear regression line is plotted on the chart, and the estimated regression line appears in the upper-corner of the chart. See the instructive video at [URL]

    https://www.youtube.com/watch?v=tnWiGyIgnV4.

4. Now perform a simple linear regression in Epi Info. Go back and select Add Analysis Gadget, Advanced Statistics, and Linear Regression. For the outcome variable, select Sigmoidoscopy and under Fields, select College. The output gives the estimated intercept and coefficient for the regression line, with corresponding statistics. For simple linear regression (i.e., one independent variable), the $F = t^2$.

5. Open Epi Info, the VISUAL DASHBOARD, and then Set Data Source. Open the Excel Workbook Application 6.3.xlsx, select Sheet1$, and click OK. Click and choose Add Analysis Gadget, Advanced Statistics, and Logistic Regression. For the Outcome Variable, select Task_Completed. For the Fields, select Quality. Make the variable Quality a dummy variable. Interpret the model.

6. Open Epi Info, the VISUAL DASHBOARD, and then Set Data Source. Open the Excel Workbook Application 6.4.xlsx, select Sheet1$, and click OK. Click and choose Add Analysis Gadget, Advanced Statistics,

and Logistic Regression. For the Outcome Variable, select Outcome. For the Fields, select Exposed. Compare the result with Practice Problem 7.

7. Open Epi Info, the VISUAL DASHBOARD, and then Set Data Source. Open the Excel Workbook Application 6.5.xlsx, select Sheet1$, and click OK. Click and choose Add Analysis Gadget, Advanced Statistics, and Linear Regression. For the Outcome Variable, select y. For the Fields, select x. Compare the result with Practice Problem 14.

8. Open Epi Info, the VISUAL DASHBOARD, and then Set Data Source. Choose the Excel Workbook Application 6.6.xlsx, select Sheet1$, and click OK. Click and choose Add Analysis Gadget, Advanced Statistics, and Linear Regression. For the Outcome Variable, select CTS (Change Total Steps). For the Fields, select TotalSteps_T1, Group, Sex, and Age. Make Group and Sex dummy variables. Sex and Age are not significant, so drop these variables and rerun the model. Note that when multiple independent variables are included in the model, estimates for each are controlled (or adjusted) for the other variables in the model. Interpret the results. Repeat the model for CBF, CBMI, and CHT. Interpret the results.

9. Open Epi Info, the VISUAL DASHBOARD, and then Set Data Source. Choose the Excel Workbook F:\Application 6.6.xlsx, select Sheet1$, and click OK. Click and choose Add Analysis Gadget, Advanced Statistics, and Logistic Regression. For the Outcome Variable, select Increased_TS. For the Fields, select TotalSteps_T1, Group, Sex, and Age. Make Group and Sex dummy variables. Sex is not significant, so drop this variable and rerun the model. Interpret the results. Repeat the model for Decreased_BF, Decreased_BMI, and Decreased_HT. Interpret the results.

10. Open the Excel workbook Application 6.7.xlsx and review how to compute Practice Problems 16 and 17.

11. In this chapter, we presented a community-based study of respiratory illness during the first year of life, which was conducted in South Carolina. Open the Excel workbook Application 6.8.xlsx and review how the odds ratios and corresponding 95% confidence intervals were computed. In Epi Info, use STATCALC and CHI SQUARE FOR TREND. What is the chi-square for linear trend value and the corresponding p-value? Interpret the result.

12. Suppose we are conducting a case-control study comparing ill and not ill individuals according to their exposure status. We want to know the sample size required for cases and controls. If we expect that 10% of controls will be exposed ($P_2 = 0.1$) and wish to detect an odds ratio of 3 with the exposure, what is the required sample size? Note that $P_1 = (OR \times P_2) / \big((1 - P_2) + (OR \times P_2)\big) = (3 \times 0.1) / \big((1 - 0.1) + (3 \times 0.1)\big) = 0.25$. With this information, the sample size can be obtained by applying the equations in Chapter 4. Alternatively, open Epi Info, the STATCALC, UNMATCHED CASE-CONTROL. Then, select a two-sided confidence level of 95%, power of 80%, ratio of controls to cases of 1, percent of controls exposed of 10%, and an odds ratio of 3. The required sample size for cases and controls is presented for three methods: Kelsey, Fleiss, and Fleiss with a continuity correction.

References

1. Doll, R., & Hill, A. B. (1966). Mortality of British doctors in relation to smoking; observations on coronary thrombosis. In W. Haenszel (Ed.), Epidemiological approaches to the study of cancer and other chronic diseases. *National Cancer Institute Monograph, 19*, 204–268.
2. The JACC study. *Am J Epidemiol, 161*(2):170–179.

Practice Problems

6.1

Calculate and interpret the risk ratio for $a = 16$, $b = 8$, $c = 6$, and $d = 20$. Express your answer to the nearest hundredth.

_____

6.2

What is the 95% confidence interval for the risk ratio computed in the last practice problem? Express your answer to the nearest hundredth.

_____ , _____

6.3

Calculate the rate ratio for $a = 16$, $b = 8$, $c = 6$, $d = 20$, $PT_e = 850$, and $PT_o = 925$. Let PT = person-years. Express your answer to the nearest hundredth.

_____

6.4

What is the 95% confidence interval for the rate ratio computed in the last practice problem? Express your answer to the nearest hundredth.

_____ , _____

6.5

What is the risk difference for 1 (per 100)? Express your answer to the nearest hundredth.

_____

What is the rate difference for 3 (per 100)? Express your answer to the nearest hundredth.

_____

6.6

Consider the data in the following table and complete the next table.

Population	Lung Cancer Incidence Rate per 100,000 Person-Years	Coronary Heart Disease (CHD) Incidence Rate per 100,000 Person-Years
Overall	$R = 60$	$R = 240$
Cigarette smokers	$R_e = 180$	$R_e = 420$
Nonsmokers	$R_o = 20$	$R_o = 180$

Population	Equation	Lung Cancer	Coronary Heart Disease (CHD)	Interpretation
RR	R_e/R_o			
AF_p	$\dfrac{R - R_o}{R} \times 100$			
	$R - R_o$ per 100,000 person-years			
AF_e	$\dfrac{R_e - R_o}{R_e} \times 100$			
	$R_e - R_o$ per 100,000 person-years			

6.7

Calculate the odds ratio for $a = 16$, $b = 8$, $c = 6$, and $d = 20$. Express your answer to the nearest hundredth.

_____

6.8

Calculate the 95% confidence interval for the odds ratio in the previous exercise. Express your answer to the nearest hundredth.

_____ , _____

6.9

Calculate AF_e when OR = 6.67.

_____ %

6.10

Calculate AF_p for the data above.

_____ %

6.11

What is the dependency ratio if 1/4 of the population is < 15 and 1/6 of the population is ≥ 65?

6.12

Calculate the t-statistic, degrees of freedom, and the p-value, given $r = 0.56$ and $n = 50$. Express your answer to the nearest hundredth.

_____

6.13

The estimated regression line for the data shown in the following table is

$$\text{Sigmoidoscopy} = 54.580 + 0.586 \times \text{College}$$

College + Adults Aged 18+ %	Sigmoidoscopy Adults Aged 50+ %	College + Adults Aged 18+ %	Sigmoidoscopy Adults Aged 50+ %
20.4	67.6	26.2	66.8
24.1	64.3	25.8	67.6
23.9	68.1	19.9	63
18.2	64.6	31	77.8
27.3	66.6	32.5	67.7
33.4	69.3	22.8	63
32.9	76.1	30.4	70.7
26.1	76.6	24.3	73.2
24.1	69.9	25	65.3
24.7	69.8	22.8	67.6
27.3	65.7	21	62.3
22.4	66.4	26.8	70.6
28.4	65.1	25.1	69.6
20.8	65	27.9	77.8
23.4	71.1	22.5	71.3
27	67.8	23.8	69.7
19.3	69.6	21.5	68.8
19.8	66.4	23.5	63.5
25.6	78.1	25.8	74.2
33.3	73	31.5	75.3
35.5	77.9	31.7	72
23.4	74.6	28.7	71.8
29.6	74.4	16.6	66
18.1	62.9	24.3	75.9
23.8	66.7	22.8	61.8

The standard error for the slope b_1 is 0.125. Calculate the following:

t statistic _____

The corresponding *p*-value _____

A 95% confidence interval for the slope estimate _____

Is there a significant relationship between education and sigmoidoscopy?

_____

6.14

Muscle mass is expected to decrease with age. Suppose you are interested in studying this relationship in a group of 20 women aged 30 through 79. You choose four women to represent each 10-year age range. Assume that a simple linear regression model is appropriate.

i	1	2	3	4	5	6	7	8	9	10
x_i	34	36	32	38	45	43	45	49	56	56
y_i	109	118	132	122	116	100	98	89	98	112
i	11	12	13	14	15	16	17	18	19	20
x_i	58	53	64	67	68	65	71	73	76	78
y_i	82	73	91	81	78	85	64	74	65	77

A. Calculate the estimated regression function. Express your answer to the nearest hundredth.

_____

B. What is a point estimate of the mean muscle mass for a woman aged 60 years? Express your answer to the nearest tenth. _____

C. What is the coefficient of determination? Express your answer to the nearest thousandth. _____

D. What is the *t*-statistic and corresponding *p*-value for evaluating whether the association between muscle mass and age is significant? Express your answer to the nearest hundredth. _____

E. What is the standard error of the slope? Express your answer to the nearest ten-thousandth. _____

F. Calculate a 95% confidence interval for the slope. Express your answer to the nearest hundredth. _____ , _____

6.15

Suppose you are interested in studying the relationship between an employee's emotional stability (X) and his or her ability to perform a task (Y). Emotional stability was determined from a questionnaire ($1 = $ Good, $0 = $ Poor), and ability to perform a task was evaluated by the supervisor ($1 = $ Yes, $0 = $ No). The results for a sample of 24 employees are:

	Task Completed	Task Not Completed
Good	7	4
Poor	5	8

The resulting slope estimate using simple logistic regression is $b_1 = 1.0295$, SE $= 0.8473$. Calculate the odds ratio and corresponding 95% confidence interval for these data. Express your answer to the nearest hundredth.

_____

_____ , _____

6.16

Consider the data in the following table, obtained from a cohort study conducted by Iso and colleagues.

Total Cardiovascular Disease According to Smoking Status

	Disease		
Current Smoker	Cases		Person-Years
Yes	882	—	220,965
No	673	—	189,254

Isa H, Date C, Yamamoto A, et al. (2005). Smoking cessation and mortality from cardiovascular disease among Japanese men and women.[2]

The resulting slope estimate using simple Poisson regression is $b_1 = 0.1155$, with a standard error SE $= 0.0512$. Calculate the rate ratio and the corresponding 95% confidence interval for these data. Express your answer to the nearest hundredth.

_____

_____ , _____

6.17

Another example is based on the study of Doll and Hill (1966), where they examined the association between death from coronary heart disease and smoking status according to age.[1] The study involved male British doctors who were followed over time using a cohort design.

Age	Smoke	Deaths	Person-Years
35–44	Yes	32	52,407
45–54	Yes	104	43,248
55–64	Yes	206	28,612
65–74	Yes	186	12,663
75–84	Yes	102	5317
35–44	No	2	18,790
45–54	No	12	10,673
55–64	No	28	5710
65–74	No	28	2585
75–84	No	31	1462

The estimated Poisson regression model is as follows:

$$\text{Death} = -7.9193 + 0.3545\,\text{Smoke} + 1.484\,\text{Age}_{45-54} + 2.6275\,\text{Age}_{55-64}$$
$$+ 3.3505\,\text{Age}_{65-74} + 3.7001\,\text{Age}_{75-84}$$

The standard errors for each of the estimates are 0.1918, 0.1074, 0.1951, 0.1837, 0.1848, and 0.1922.

Calculate the rate ratio for each of the slope estimates and their corresponding 95% confidence intervals. Express your answers to the nearest hundredth.

	Rate Ratio	95% Confidence Interval
35–44	1.00	—
45–54		
55–64		
65–74		
75–84		
Nonsmoker		
Smoker		

Appendix A

Notation and Equations

▶ Notation

Capital letters are typically used to represent population attributes (parameters), and lowercase letters represent sample attributes (statistics). For example,

- X_i = the ith observation in a population; x_i = the ith observation in a sample
- N = the number of observations in a population; n = the number of observations in a sample

Greek letters are used to represent population attributes (parameters), and Roman letters are used to represent sample attributes (statistics). For example,

- μ refers to a population mean; $\bar{x}$ refers to a sample mean.
- σ refers to the standard deviation of a population; s refers to the standard deviation of a sample.
- β refers to the population slope coefficient; b refers to the sample slope coefficient.
- ρ refers to the population correlation coefficient; r refers to the sample correlation coefficient.
- π (or P) refers to a population proportion; p = a sample proportion.
- There is not a symbol for the population parameter of the median, but the sample statistic is represented as $\bar{x}$.

▶ Probability

- An event is one or more outcomes of an experiment. Consider two events, A and B.
- $0 \leq A \leq 1, 0 \leq B \leq 1$.
- $P(A)$ refers to the probability that event A will occur.
- If A and B occur together, then $P(A \text{ or } B) = P(A) + P(B) - P(A \text{ and } B)$.
- If A and B are mutually exclusive (they cannot both occur at the same time), then $P(A \text{ or } B) = P(A) + P(B)$.
- $P(A \mid B) = P(A \text{ and } B)/P(B)$ refers to the probability that event A will occur, given that event B has occurred.
- If events A and B are independent (i.e., the occurrence of one does not influence the probability of the other occurring), then $P(A \text{ and } B) = P(A)P(B)$.
- Bayes' Theorem is used to compute posterior probabilities from prior and observed probabilities. For events A and B, provided $P(B) \neq 0$, $P(A \mid B) = P(B \mid A)P(A)/P(B)$.
- $E(X)$ is the expected value of the random variable X.
- $P(X = x \mid n, p)$ refers to binomial probability.

- $P(X = x \mid \mu)$ refers to Poisson probability.
- $n!$ refers to the factorial value of n.

▶ Hypothesis Testing

- H_0 refers to a null hypothesis.
- H_a refers to an alternative hypothesis.
- α refers to the level of significance; the probability of a Type I error.
- β refers to the probability of committing a Type II error.
- Power $= 1 - \beta$.
- γ refers to the confidence coefficient $(1 - \alpha)$. The confidence level is $(1 - \alpha)100\%$.

▶ Special Symbols

Certain symbols have special meanings. For example:

- f_i = frequency of X_i.
- f = total number of observations in an interval.
- $f(x)$ refers to a probability density function.
- Σ is the summation symbol, used to compute sums over a range of values.
- $\displaystyle\sum_{i}^{n} x_i$ refers to the sum of a set of n observations. Thus, $\displaystyle\sum_{i}^{n} x_i = x_1 + x_2 + \cdots + x_n$.
- *sqrt* refers to the square root function.
- $\text{Var}(X)$ refers to the variance of the random variable X.
- $\text{SD}(X)$ refers to the standard deviation of the random variable X.
- SE refers to the standard error of a statistic.
- ME refers to the margin of error.
- df refers to the degrees of freedom.
- $|x|$ is the absolute value of X.
- $\approx$ is approximately equal.

▶ Selected Formulas and Equations

Mean

$$\mu = \sum_{i=1}^{N} \frac{X_i}{N} = \frac{1}{N} \sum_{i=1}^{N} X_i$$

$$\bar{x} = \sum_{i=1}^{n} \frac{x_i}{n} = \frac{1}{n} \sum_{i=1}^{n} x_i$$

$$\bar{x} = \sum_{i=1}^{n} f_i \frac{x_i}{n} = \frac{1}{n} \sum_{i=1}^{n} f_i x_i$$

$$GM = \sqrt[n]{(X_1)(X_2)\ldots(X_n)}$$

Variance

$$\sigma^2 = \frac{1}{N} \sum_{i=1}^{N} (X_i - \mu)^2$$

$$s^2 = \frac{1}{n-1} \sum_{i=1}^{n} (x_i - \bar{x})^2$$

$$s^2 = \frac{1}{\left(\sum_{i=1}^{n} f_i - 1\right)} \sum_{i=1}^{n} f_i (x_i - \bar{X})^2$$

Standard Deviation

$$\sigma = \sqrt{\sigma^2} = \sqrt{\frac{1}{N} \sum_{i=1}^{N} (X_i - \mu)^2}$$

$$s = \sqrt{s^2} = \sqrt{\frac{1}{n-1} \sum_{i=1}^{n} (x_i - \bar{X})^2}$$

$$s = \sqrt{s^2} = \sqrt{\frac{1}{\left(\sum_{i=1}^{n} f_i - 1\right)} \sum_{i=1}^{n} f_i (x_i - \bar{X})^2}$$

Standard Error (SE) of the Mean

$$SE = \sigma_\mu = \frac{\sigma}{\sqrt{N}}$$

$$SE = s_{\bar{x}} = \frac{s}{\sqrt{n}}$$

Finite Population Correction Factor

$$\sqrt{\frac{N-n}{N-1}}$$

Coefficient of Variation

$$CV = \frac{\sigma}{\mu} \times 100$$

$$CV = \frac{s}{\bar{x}} \times 100$$

▶ Measures of Validity

$$\text{Sensitivity} = \frac{\text{TP}}{\text{TP} + \text{FN}}$$

$$\text{Specificity} = \frac{\text{TN}}{\text{FP} + \text{TN}}$$

$$\text{Predictive Value} = \frac{\text{TP}}{\text{TP} + \text{FP}}$$

$$\text{Predictive Value} = \frac{\text{TN}}{\text{FN} + \text{TN}}$$

▶ Equations for Confidence Intervals

$$L = \bar{X} - Z_{\propto/2}\frac{\sigma}{\sqrt{n}} \text{ and } R = \bar{X} + Z_{\propto/2}\frac{\sigma}{\sqrt{n}}$$

$$L = \bar{X} - t_{n-1,\propto/2}\frac{s}{\sqrt{n}} \text{ and } R = \bar{X} + t_{n-1,\propto/2}\frac{s}{\sqrt{n}}$$

$$L = \bar{d} - t_{n-1,\propto/2}\frac{s_d}{\sqrt{n}} \text{ and } R = \bar{d} + t_{n-1,\propto/2}\frac{s_d}{\sqrt{n}}$$

$$L = (\bar{X}_1 - \bar{X}_2) - t_{n_1+n_2-2,\propto/2}\text{SE}_{(\bar{X}_1-\bar{X}_2)} \text{ and } R = (\bar{X}_1 - \bar{X}_2) - t_{n_1+n_2-2,\propto/2}\text{SE}_{(\bar{X}_1-\bar{X}_2}$$

$$L = \text{Rate} - t_{n_1+n_2-2,\propto/2}\sqrt{\frac{\text{Rate}(1 - \text{Rate})}{\text{Population at risk}}} \text{ and}$$

$$R = \text{Rate} + t_{n_1+n_2-2,\propto/2}\sqrt{\frac{\text{Rate}(1 - \text{Rate})}{\text{Population at risk}}}$$

▶ Pooled Standard Deviation

$$s_p = \sqrt{\frac{(n_1 - 1)s_1^2 + (n_2 - 1)s_2^2}{n_1 + n_2 - 2}}$$

▶ Standard Error of the Difference

$$\text{SE}_{(\bar{X}_1-\bar{X}_2)} = s_p\sqrt{\frac{1}{n_1} + \frac{1}{n_2}}$$

t-Test for Comparing Means

$$t_{n_1+n_2-2} = \frac{(\bar{X}_1 - \bar{X}_2) - 0}{\text{SE}_{(\bar{X}_1-\bar{X}_2)}}$$

If Variances Are Significantly Different

$$t_v = \frac{(\bar{X}_1 - \bar{X}_2) - 0}{\sqrt{(s_1^2 / n_1) + (s_2^2 / n_2)}} \qquad v = \frac{\left[(s_1^2 / n_1) + (s_2^2 / n_2)\right]^2}{\left[(s_1^2 / n_1)^2 / (n_1 - 1) + (s_2^2 / n_2)^2 / (n_2 - 1)\right]}$$

▶ Equation for the Chi-Square for a Contingency Table

$$\chi^2 = \sum_i \sum_j \frac{(n_{ij} - m_{ij})^2}{m_{ij}}$$

where $m_{ij} = R_i C_j / n$

▶ Computational Formulas for One-Way ANOVA

Source of Variation	Sums of Squares	Degrees of Freedom	Mean Squares	F-Test Statistic
Among	$SS_A = \sum (X_j - \bar{\bar{X}})^2 = \sum n_j \bar{X}_j^2 - \frac{\left(\sum X_{ij}\right)^2}{N}$	$j - 1$	$MS_A = \frac{SS_A}{j - 1}$	$F = \frac{MS_A}{MS_w}$
Within	$SS_W = SS_T - SS_A$	$N - j$	$MS_W = \frac{SS_W}{N - j}$	
Total	$SS_T = \sum (X_{ij} - \bar{\bar{X}})^2 = \sum X_{ij}^2 - \frac{\left(\sum X_{ij}\right)^2}{N}$	$N - 1$		

▶ Calculating the Correlation Coefficient for a Sample

$$r = \frac{\sum (x - \bar{x})(y - \bar{y})}{\sqrt{\sum (x - \bar{x})^2 (y - \bar{y})^2}}$$

t-Distribution with *n* − 2 Degrees of Freedom for Assessing ρ

$$t = \frac{r\sqrt{n - 2}}{\sqrt{1 - r^2}}$$

▶ # Calculating the Spearman Rho

$$r = \frac{\sum (R_X - \bar{R}_X)(R_Y - \bar{R}_Y)}{\sqrt{\sum (R_X - \bar{R}_X)^2 (R_Y - \bar{R}_Y)^2}}$$

▶ # Simple Regression

$$Y = \beta_0 + \beta_1 X + \epsilon$$

For a data set (x_i, y_i), where $(\bar{x}, \bar{y})$ are the centroids (means) and r is the correlation coefficient:

$e_i = y_i - \hat{y}_i$ (Residuals)
$\hat{y}_i = b_0 + b_1 x_i$ (Least squares regression line; $\hat{y}_i$ represents the predicted value of Y)

$$\text{SSM} = \sum (\bar{y} - \hat{y}_i)^2 \cdot \text{SSE} = \sum (y_i - \hat{y}_i)^2 \cdot \text{SST} = \text{SSM} + \text{SSE}$$

$r^2 = \text{SSM/SST}$ (Coefficient of determination)
$\text{MSE} = \text{SSE}/(n-2)$ (Unbiased estimator of σ^2)

$$b_1 = \sum (x - \bar{x})(y - \bar{y}) / \sum (x - \bar{x})^2 \text{ (Least-squares estimate of } \beta_1)$$

$$b_1 = r \frac{s_x}{s_y}$$

$$b_0 = \bar{y} - b_1 \bar{x} \text{ (Least-squares estimate of } \beta_0)$$

$$\text{SE}_{b_1} = \sqrt{\frac{1/(n-2) \sum (y_i - \hat{y}_i)^2}{\sum (x_i - \bar{x})^2}}$$

$$\text{SE}_{b_0} = s \sqrt{\frac{1}{n} + \frac{\bar{x}^2}{\sum (x_i - \bar{x})^2}}$$

$$s = \sqrt{\text{MSE}} = \sqrt{\frac{\text{SSE}}{n-2}}$$

$b_1 \pm t_{n-1, \propto/2} \text{SE}_{b_1}$ (Confidence interval for the slope, β_1)
$b_0 \pm t_{n-1, \propto/2} \text{SE}_{b_0}$ (Confidence interval for the intercept, β_0)
$\hat{y}_h \pm t_{n-1, \propto/2} s \sqrt{1 + (1/n)} + (x_h - \bar{x})^2 / \sum (x_i - \bar{x})^2$ (Prediction limits for a new observation Y given at x_h)
$t = (b_1 - \beta_1) / \text{SE}_{b_1}$ (t-statistic for testing the significance of the slope)

▶ # Multiple Regression Model

$$Y = \beta_0 + \beta_1 X_1 + \beta_2 X_2 + \cdots + \beta_k X_k + \epsilon$$
$$\hat{y} = b_0 + b_1 x_1 + b_2 x_2 + \cdots + b_k x_k$$
$$Y = X\beta + \epsilon \text{ (Matrix form)}$$

Where there are n observed values of Y and n associated observed values for each of k different X variables:

$$Y = \begin{bmatrix} Y_1 \\ \vdots \\ Y_n \end{bmatrix}, X = \begin{bmatrix} 1X_{11} & \cdots & X_{1k} \\ \vdots & \ddots & \vdots \\ 1X_{n1} & \cdots & X_{nk} \end{bmatrix}, \beta = \begin{bmatrix} \beta_0 \\ \vdots \\ \beta_n \end{bmatrix}, \epsilon = \begin{bmatrix} \epsilon_1 \\ \vdots \\ \epsilon_n \end{bmatrix}$$

$b = (X'X)^{-1}X'Y$ (Least-squares estimate of the column vector β)

$\hat{y} = Xb$ (Estimated regression model)

▶ Natural Logarithm

The natural logarithm is used in this book to obtain estimated annual percent change, odds ratios, rate ratios, and hazard ratios from regression models. The letter e is the base used in natural logarithms. It is the limiting value of the expression $e = 2.718 = (1 + (1 / x))^x$ as $x \to \infty$. The natural logarithm y using base e is $\ln(y)$. Some properties of logarithms are expressed in the following table:

Properties of Logarithms	
	Formula
Product	$\ln(xy) = \ln(x) + \ln(y)$
Quotient	$\ln(x/y) = \ln(x) - \ln(y)$
Power	$\ln(x^p) = p\ln(x)$
Root	$\ln\sqrt[p]{x} = \dfrac{\ln(x)}{p}$

▶ Proportion

$$\pi = \frac{X}{N}$$

X is the number of successes

$$p = \frac{x}{n}$$

$$SE_p = \sqrt{\frac{p(1 - p)}{n}}$$

$$p \pm Z_{\alpha/2}SE_p$$

$$Z = \frac{p - \pi_0}{SE_p}$$

$$SE_{p_1 - p_2} = \sqrt{\frac{p_1(1 - p_1)}{n_1} + \frac{p_2(1 - p_2)}{n_2}}$$

$$(p_1 - p_2) \pm Z_{\infty/2}\text{SE}_{p_1 - p_2}$$

If $\pi_1 = \pi_2$, then we can pool the variances and reduce the variance:

$$p_{\text{pooled}} = \frac{x_1 + x_2}{n_1 + n_2}$$

$$\text{SE}_{p_1 - p_2} = \sqrt{p_{\text{pooled}}(1 - p_{\text{pooled}})\left[\frac{1}{n_1} + \frac{1}{n_2}\right]}$$

$$Z = \frac{p_1 - p_2}{\text{SE}_{p_1 - p_2}}$$

Z has an approximate standard normal distribution if n_1 and n_2 are large.

▶ Logistic Regression Model

$$\pi = \beta_0 + \beta_1 X + \epsilon$$

$$\ln(\text{Odds}) = \ln\left[\frac{\pi}{1 - \pi}\right] = \beta_0 + \beta_1 X + \epsilon$$

$$\ln(\text{Odds}) = \ln\left[\frac{p}{1 - p}\right] = b_0 + b_1 x$$

$$\ln(\text{Odds})_{\text{Exposed}} = b_0 + b_1 \times 1$$

$$\ln(\text{Odds})_{\text{Unexposed}} = b_0 + b_1 \times 0$$

$$b_1 = \ln(\text{Odds})_{\text{Exposed}} - \ln(\text{Odds})_{\text{Unexposed}} = \ln(\text{Odds ratio})$$

$$\text{Odds ratio} = e^{b_1}$$

▶ Multiple Logistic Regression Model

$$\ln(\text{Odds}) = \beta_0 + \beta_1 X_1 + \beta_2 X_2 + \cdots + \beta_k X_k + \epsilon$$

$$\ln(\text{Odds}) = b_0 + b_1 x_1 + b_2 x_2 + \cdots + b_k x_k$$

▶ Poisson Regression

$$\ln(\text{Rate})_{\text{Exposed}} = b_0 + b_1 \times 1$$

$$\ln(\text{Rate})_{\text{Unexposed}} = b_0 + b_1 \times 0$$

$$b_1 = \ln(\text{Rate})_{\text{Exposed}} - \ln(\text{Rate})_{\text{Unexposed}} = \ln(\text{Rate ratio})$$

$$\text{Rate ratio} = e^{b_1}$$

▶ 2 × 2 Table Where the Letters Represent Numbers

	Cases	Controls	Total
Exposed	a	b	$a + b$
Not Exposed	c	d	$c + d$
Total	$a + c$	$b + d$	$n = a + b + c + d$

▶ Odds Ratio

$$\text{OR} = \frac{P(\text{Exposed}\,|\,\text{Disease})\,/\,P(\text{Unexposed}\,|\,\text{Disease})}{P(\text{Exposed}\,|\,\text{No disease})\,/\,P(\text{Unexposed}\,|\,\text{No disease})} = \frac{a\,/\,c}{b\,/\,d} = \frac{a \times c}{b \times d}$$

▶ Risk Ratio

$$\text{Risk ratio} = \frac{P(\text{Outcome}\,|\,\text{Exposed})}{P(\text{Outcome}\,|\,\text{Not exposed})}$$

$$= \frac{a\,/\,(a + b)}{c\,/\,(c + d)} = \frac{\text{Attack rate for exposed}}{\text{Attack rate for not exposed}}$$

$$\text{RR}_{\text{MH}} = \frac{\sum\left(a_i[c_i + d_i]\,/\,n_i\right)}{\sqrt{\sum\left(c_i[a_i + b_i]\,/\,n_i\right)}}$$

▶ Rate Ratio

$$\text{Rate ratio} = \frac{P(\text{Outcome}\,|\,\text{Exposed})}{P(\text{Outcome}\,|\,\text{Not exposed})} = \frac{a\,/\,\text{PT}_e}{c\,/\,\text{PT}_o}$$

$$= \frac{\text{Person–time rate for exposed}}{\text{Person–time rate for not exposed}}$$

▶ Prevalence Ratio

$$\text{PR} = \frac{P(\text{Outcome}\,|\,\text{Exposed})}{P(\text{Outcome}\,|\,\text{Not exposed})} = \frac{a\,/\,(a + b)}{c\,/\,(c + d)}$$

Appendix B

Answers to Odd-Numbered Practice Problems

▶ Chapter 2

2.1

Answer:

$-5 > -10$
$a \geq 0$
$-2 < b < -1$
$c < 5 \leq d$

For more information, see Chapter 2, Number Line.

2.3

Answer:

π
2
5
$20\pi - 2\pi^2$ or 43

For more information, see Chapter 2, Properties (or Laws) of Arithmetic and Algebraic Operations.

2.5

Possible answer: $-5 - 3 = -8$, but $3 - (-5) = 3 + 5 = 8$

For more information, see Chapter 2, Properties (or Laws) of Arithmetic and Algebraic Operations.

2.7

Possible answer: $(10 - 5) - 2 = 5 - 2 = 3$, but $10 - (5 - 2) = 10 - 3 = 7$

For more information, see Chapter 2, Properties (or Laws) of Arithmetic and Algebraic Operations.

2.9

Answer: $x = 3, x = 2$

Further description: The zero product property says:

If $(x - 3)(x - 2) = 0$ then $(x - 3) = 0$ or $(x - 2) = 0$

For $(x - 3) = 0$ we get $x = 3$
For $(x - 2) = 0$ we get $x = 2$
For more information, see Chapter 2, Properties (or Laws) of Arithmetic and Algebraic Operations.

2.11

Answer: 4

For more information, see Chapter 2, Properties (or Laws) of Arithmetic and Algebraic Operations.

2.13

Answer: 14

Further description:

$$\frac{1}{8} + \frac{1}{33} - \frac{1}{12} = \frac{396 + 96 - 264}{3168} = \frac{228}{3168} = \frac{1}{14}$$

There is a net gain of one person every 14 s.
For more information, see Chapter 2, Fractions.

2.15

1.33, 33

Further description:

$$\frac{1 / 6}{1 / 8} = \frac{1}{1} \times \frac{8}{6} = \frac{8}{6} = \frac{4}{3} = 1.33$$

So the lifetime risk of prostate cancer in men is 1.33 times (or 33%) greater than the lifetime risk of breast cancer in women.
For more information, see Chapter 2, Fractions.

2.17

A. $2^3 2^4 = 128 = 2^{3+4} = 2^7$

B. $\dfrac{2^3}{2^4} = \dfrac{1}{2} = 2^{3-4} = 2^{-1}$

C. $(2^3)^4 = 4096 = 2^{3\times 4} = 2^{12}$

D. $(2 \times 5)^4 = 10000 = 2^4 5^4$

E. $\left(\dfrac{2}{5}\right)^4 = 0.4^4 = 0.0256 = \dfrac{2^4}{5^4} = \dfrac{16}{625}$

F. $\dfrac{1}{2^{-4}} = \dfrac{1}{0.065} = 16 = 2^4$

For more information, see Chapter 2, Exponents and Roots.

2.19

Answer:

Rank	Name	2015	2016	r
1	Utah	2,990,632	3,051,217	0.0203
2	Nevada	2,883,758	2,940,058	0.0195
3	Idaho	1,652,828	1,683,140	0.0183
4	Florida	20,244,914	20,612,439	0.0182
5	Washington	7,160,290	7,288,000	0.0178
6	Oregon	4,024,634	4,093,465	0.0171
7	Colorado	5,448,819	5,540,545	0.0168
8	Arizona	6,817,565	6,931,071	0.0166
9	District of Columbia	670,377	681,170	0.0161
10	Texas	27,429,639	27,862,596	0.0158

Source: https://www.census.gov/newsroom/press-releases/2016/cb16-214.html

For more information, see Chapter 2, Exponential Functions.

2.21

Answer: 6,084,475

Further description:

$$y = f(x) = ae^{rt} = 3,051,217e^{0.0203 \times 34} = 6,084,475$$

For more information, see Chapter 2, Exponential Functions.

2.23

Answer:

Logarithmic form	
$\log_a y = x$	$y = a^x$
$\log_3 9 = 2$	$9 = 3^2$
$\log_3 27 = 3$	$27 = 3^3$
$\log_4 \dfrac{1}{16} = -2$	$\dfrac{1}{16} = 4^{-2}$

▶ Chapter 3

3.1

Answer:

66
44

Number of Children	Frequency	Relative Frequency	Cumulative Frequency	Cumulative Relative Frequency
0	8	0.16	8	0.16
1	11	0.22	19	0.38
2	14	0.28	33	0.66
3	8	0.16	41	0.82
4	5	0.10	46	0.92
5+	4	0.08	50	1

For more information, see Chapter 3, Descriptive Measures: Nominal and Ordinal Data.

3.3

Answer: 61.9 per 100
Further description:

$$\frac{78}{126} \times 10^2 = 61.9 \text{ per } 100$$

For more information, see Chapter 3, Descriptive Measures: Nominal and Ordinal Data.

3.5

Answer: 25 per 100
Further description:

$$\frac{120}{480} \times 10^2 = 25.0 \text{ per } 100$$

3.7

Answer: 23%
Further description:

$$\frac{120 - 20}{480 - 20} \times 10^2 = 21.7 \text{ per } 100$$

For more information, see Chapter 3, Descriptive Measures: Nominal and Ordinal Data.

3.9

Answer:

Crude mortality rate	882 per 100,000
Maternal mortality rate	154 per 100,000
Infant mortality rate	28 per 1,000
Neonatal mortality rate	15 per 1,000
Post neonatal mortality rate	12 per 1,000
Fetal death rate	20 per 1,000
Fertility rate	72 per 1,000
Age-specific mortality rate for persons aged 55 years or older	18 per 1,000
Cause-specific mortality rate for heart disease	82 per 100,000
Cause-specific mortality rate for stroke	35 per 100,000
Proportional mortality ratio for cancer among persons ages 55 years or older	5 per 100
Death-to-Case Ratio for heart disease	26 per 100
Abortion rate	55 per 1,000
Rate of natural increase	10 per 1,000

For more information, see Chapter 3, Descriptive Measures: Nominal and Ordinal Data.

3.11

Answer: 5.66

Further description:

$$\text{GM} = \sqrt[16]{(1^1)(2^2)(4^4)(8^6)(16^3)} = 5.66$$

For more information, see Chapter 3, Descriptive Measures: Numerical Data.

3.13

Answer:

0–4	2.5
5–9	7.5
10–14	12.5
15–19	17.5
20–24	22.5
25–29	27.5

For more information, see Chapter 3, Descriptive Measures: Numerical Data.

▶ Chapter 4

4.1

Answer: 0.454

Further description:

$$P(\text{Local stage}) = 0.454$$

For more information, see Chapter 4, Probability Concepts.

4.3

Answer:

0.473
0.369
0.417
0.438

Further description:

$$P(\text{Local stage} \mid \text{White}) = \frac{0.355}{0.751} = 0.473$$

$$P(\text{Local stage} \mid \text{Black}) = \frac{0.052}{0.141} = 0.369$$

$$P(\text{Local stage} \mid \text{AI or AN}) = \frac{0.005}{0.012} = 0.417$$

$$P(\text{Local stage} \mid \text{A or PI}) = \frac{0.042}{0.096} = 0.438$$

For more information, see Chapter 4, Probability Concepts.

4.5

Answer: 0.850

Further description:

$$P(\text{Local stage or White}) = P(\text{Local stage}) + P(\text{White}) - P(\text{Local stage and white})$$
$$= 0.454 + 0.751 - 0.355 = 0.850$$

For more information, see Chapter 4, Probability Concepts.

4.7

Answer:

1.20
1.69
1.06

Further description:

$$\frac{P(\text{Distant} \mid \text{Black})}{P(\text{Distant} \mid \text{White})} = \frac{0.025 \,/\, 0.141}{0.111 \,/\, 0.751} = 1.20.$$

Therefore, among cervical cancer patients, black women are 1.20 (or 20%) more likely than whites to be diagnosed with distant staged disease.

$$\frac{P(\text{Cervical cancer} \mid \text{American Indian...})}{P(\text{Cervical cancer} \mid \text{White})} = \frac{0.003 \,/\, 0.012}{0.111 \,/\, 0.751} = 1.69.$$

Therefore, among cervical cancer patients, American Indian women are 1.69 (or 69%) more likely than whites to be diagnosed with distant staged disease.

$$\frac{P(\text{Cervical cancer} \mid \text{Asian}\ldots)}{P(\text{Cervical cancer} \mid \text{White})} = \frac{0.015 \,/\, 0.096}{0.111 \,/\, 0.751} = 1.06.$$

Therefore, among cervical cancer patients, Asian women are 1.06 (or 6%) more likely than whites to be diagnosed with distant staged disease.

For more information, see Chapter 4, Probability Concepts.

4.9

Answer: 0.80

Further description:

$$\text{Specificity} = \frac{628}{783} = 0.80$$

Of those without the disease, 80% test negative.

For more information, see Chapter 4, Probability Concepts.

4.11

Answer: 0.98

Further description:

$$\text{Predictive value negative} = \frac{628}{640} = 0.98$$

Of those who test negative, 98% do not have the disease.

For more information, see Chapter 4, Probability Concepts.

4.13

Answer: 4

Further description:

$$\binom{4}{3} = \frac{4!}{3!} = \frac{4 \times 3 \times 2 \times 1}{3 \times 2 \times 1} = \frac{24}{6} = 4$$

For more information, see Chapter 4, Probability Sampling.

4.15

Answer:

$1000/100 = 10$, so every 10th person in the sample should be systematically selected. Let's first randomly select a number from 1 to 10, and then choose every 10th person thereafter.

For more information, see Chapter 4, Probability Sampling.

4.17

Answer: 0.229

$$\frac{8}{35} = 0.229$$

For more information, see Chapter 4, Probability Distribution.

4.19

Answer: 113.1, 126.9

For more information, see Chapter 4, Point Estimates for Confidence Intervals.

4.21

Answer: 131, 153

Further description:

$$0.00131, 0.00153 \rightarrow 131 - 153 \, \text{per} \, 100,000$$

For more information, see Chapter 4, Point Estimates for Confidence Intervals.

▶ Chapter 5

5.1

Answer:
0.4082
0.9082
0.0918
For more information, see Chapter 5, Hypothesis Testing.

5.3

Answer:
1.96
1.96
For more information, see Chapter 5, Hypothesis Testing.

5.5

Answer: 0.95
For more information, see Chapter 5, Hypothesis Testing.

5.7

Answer:
0.025
Reject
Further description: In the body of the t table we first locate this value. Then, going to the top of the table we find the corresponding p value, which is 0.025 (100 − 97.50). Since this value is less than 0.05, we reject H_0.
For more information, see Chapter 5, Hypothesis Testing.

5.9

Answer:

1. $H_0 : \mu = 8$
2. $H_a : \mu \neq 8$
3. $\alpha = 0.05, n = 126$
4. t-statistic and $(126 - 1) = 125$ degrees of freedom. From a t-table, the critical value is 1.97.
5. $t = \dfrac{9.5 - 8}{8 \, / \, \sqrt{126}} = 2.10$

6. The *t* statistic is above the critical value, so we reject H_0 and conclude that mean is significantly greater than 8.

What is the *p* value?

$$0.02 < p < 0.05$$

For more information, see Chapter 5, Hypothesis Testing.

5.11

Answer:

1. $H_0: \pi \geq 0.7$
2. $H_a: \pi < 0.7$
3. $\alpha = 0.05, n = 136$
4. Z statistic.
5. $z = \dfrac{f - \pi_0}{\sqrt{\pi_0(1 - \pi_0) / n}} = \dfrac{0.62 - 0.7}{\sqrt{0.7(1 - 0.7) / 136}} = -2.04$
6. The critical value is -1.645. Since $-2.04 < -1.645$, reject H_0 and conclude that the cash incentive is not sufficient to obtain at least 70% of people in the population of interest to participate.

What is the *p* value?

$$0.01 < p < 0.025$$

For more information, see Chapter 5, Hypothesis Testing.

5.13

Answer: 0.76

Further description:

$$K = \frac{2(34 \times 54 - 4 \times 8)}{30 \times 58 + 70 \times 42} = 0.76$$

Hence, there is excellent agreement between the two specialists in diagnosing SD among voice patients.

For more information, see Chapter 5, Hypothesis Testing.

5.15

Answer:

1. $H_0: \pi_1 = \pi_2$
2. $H_a: \pi_1 \neq \pi_2$
3. $\alpha = 0.05, n = 250$
4. χ^2 test with degrees of freedom $= (r - 1)(c - 1) = (2 - 1)(2 - 1) = 1$.
5. $\chi^2 = \dfrac{\left(|ad - bc| - n / 2\right)^2 n}{(a + b)(c + d)(a + c)(b + d)}$

$= \dfrac{\left(|31 \times 109 - 94 \times 16| - 250 / 2\right)^2 250}{(31 + 94)(16 + 109)(31 + 16)(94 + 109)} = 5.14$
6. The critical value is 3.84. Because $5.14 > 3.84$, we reject H_0 and conclude that those with OSA are more likely to have a voice disorder.

What is the *p* value?

$$0.025 > p > 0.01$$

For more information, see Chapter 5, Hypothesis Testing.

5.17

Answer:

1. $H_0 : \pi \geq 0.7$
2. $H_a : \pi < 0.7$
3. Assumed truth is 0.60
4. The proportion itself determines the estimated standard deviation
5. $\alpha = 0.05$ and $\beta = 0.20$.

6. $n = \left[\dfrac{1.645\sqrt{0.70(1 - 0.70)} - (-0.842)\sqrt{0.60(1 - 0.60)}}{0.70 - 0.60} \right]^2 = 136$

   Hence, the required sample size is 136.
   For more information, see Chapter 5, Sample Size.

5.19

Answer:

1. $H_0 : \pi_1 = \pi_2$
2. $H_a : \pi_1 \neq \pi_2$
3. Difference between 15% and 30%
4. The null hypothesis assumes the proportions are equal. The proportion itself determines the estimated standard deviation
5. $\alpha = 0.05$ and $\beta = 0.20$
6. $\pi = (0.15 + 0.30)/2 = 0.225$

7. $n = \left[\dfrac{1.96\sqrt{2 \times 0.225(1 - 0.225)} - (-0.842)\sqrt{0.15(1 - 0.15) + 0.30(1 - 0.30)}}{0.15 - 0.30} \right]^2$

   $= 120.5 \approx 121$ per group

   For more information, see Chapter 5, Sample Size.

5.21

Answer: 246
   Further description:

$$n = \frac{4 \times 1.96 \times 0.8 \times (1 - 0.8)}{0.1^2} = 246$$

For more information, see Chapter 5, Sample Size.

▶ Chapter 6

6.1

Answer: 2.89
   Further description:

$$\text{Risk ratio} = \frac{16 / (16 + 8)}{6 / (6 + 20)} = \frac{16 / 24}{6 / 26} = 2.89$$

Thus, those exposed are 2.89 times more likely to develop the outcome than those not exposed. We can also say that the exposed are 189% ($[2.89 - 1] \times 100$), more likely to develop the outcome as those not exposed. Note that we subtract 1 because this is the value where no association exists.

For more information, see Chapter 6, Measures of Association.

6.3

Answer: 2.90

Further description:

$$\text{Rate ratio} = \frac{16 \: / \: 850}{6 \: / \: 925} = 2.90$$

For more information, see Chapter 6, Measures of Association.

6.5

Answer: 43.59, 1.23

Further description:

$$\text{Risk difference} = \left(\frac{16}{24} - \frac{6}{26} \right) \times 100 = 43.59 \text{ per } 100$$

$$\text{Rate difference} = \left(\frac{16}{850} - \frac{6}{925} \right) \times 100 = 1.23 \text{ per } 100 \text{ person-years}$$

For more information, see Chapter 6, Measures of Association.

6.7

Answer: 6.67

Further description:

$$\text{Odds ratio} = \frac{16 \times 20}{6 \times 8} = \frac{320}{48} = \frac{20}{3} = 6.67$$

For more information, see Chapter 6, Measures of Association.

6.9

Answer: 85%

Further description:

$$\text{AF}_\text{e} = \frac{6.67 - 1}{6.67} \times 100 = 85.0\%$$

For more information, see Chapter 6, Measures of Association.

6.11

Answer: 71

Further description:

$$\frac{(1 \: / \: 4) + (1 \: / \: 6)}{1 - ([1 \: / \: 4] + [1 \: / \: 6])} \times 100 = \frac{(3 \: / \: 12) + (2 \: / \: 12)}{(12 \: / \: 12) - ([3 \: / \: 12] + [2 \: / \: 12])} \times 100$$

$$= \frac{5 \: / \: 12}{(12 \: / \: 12) - (5 \: / \: 12)} \times 100$$

$$= \frac{(5 \: / \: 12)}{(7 \: / \: 12)} \times 100 = \frac{5 \times 12}{7 \times 12} \times 100$$

$$= \frac{5}{7} \times 100 \approx 71$$

Hence there are 71 dependents for every 100 people of working age.
For more information, see Chapter 6, Measures of Association.

6.13

Answer: 4.68, $p < 0.0001$, 0.340, 0.831, Yes
    Further description:
    $t = 4.68$, $p < 0.0001$, 95% CI: $0.340 - 0.831$. So, we reject the null hypothesis of no association and conclude that education is positively associated with sigmoidoscopy.
    For more information, see Chapter 6, Numerical Data.

6.15

Answer: 2.80, 0.53, 14.73
    Further description:
    What do you conclude about statistical significance?

$$\text{Odds ratio} = e^{b_1} = e^{1.0295} = 2.8$$

$$95\% \text{ CI} : e^{1.0295 \pm 1.96 \times 0.8473} \rightarrow 0.532, 14.734$$

Because the confidence interval overlaps 1, there is not a significant association between emotional stability and completing the task.
    For more information, see Chapter 6, Numerical Data.

6.17

Answer:

	Rate Ratio	95% Confidence Interval
35–44	1.00	–
45–54	4.41	3.57, 5.44
55–64	13.8	9.44, 20.29
65–74	28.5	19.89, 40.88
75–84	40.5	28.16, 58.11
Nonsmoker	1.00	–
Smoker	1.43	0.98, 2.08

After adjusting for age, smokers have 1.43 times the mortality rate of nonsmokers. The confidence interval overlaps 1, indicating insignificance at the 0.05 level. Compared with the age group 35–44, each age has a successively significantly greater rate of death.
    For more information, see Chapter 6, Numerical Data.

Glossary

Algebra A part of mathematics that uses letters or other symbols to represent numbers that are either unknown or that can assume many values, according to the rules of arithmetic.

Alternative (or research) hypothesis A hypothesis is a proposed explanation for a phenomenon in one or more populations that can be tested by investigation. The alternative hypothesis gives the opposing opinion or conclusion to that of the null hypothesis. The goal is usually to provide sufficient evidence to support this hypothesis.

Analytic methods In epidemiology, these are techniques that allow us to search for causes and effects (i.e., address the why and how); techniques involved in measuring associations between variables and testing hypotheses of association.

Analysis of variance (ANOVA) The process of testing the hypothesis of equality of three or more means taken from j independent groups.

Arithmetic The study of numbers, particularly operations between numbers. Basic operations of arithmetic include addition, subtraction, multiplication, and division.

Attribute data Specifies characteristics of that location (e.g., city names, type of road, temperature, rainfall, address); information combined with spatial features.

Cluster sample A form of probability sample where respondents are drawn from a random sample of mutually exclusive groups (clusters) within a total population. Cluster sampling may be less expensive and more convenient than simple random sampling.

Coefficient of determination The correlation coefficient squared (denoted as r^2). This measure represents the proportion of the total variation in the outcome variable y that is determined by the exposure variable x. If $r = 1$, then all of the variation in the outcome variable is explained by the exposure variable. However, typically only part of the variation in the outcome variable will be explained by a single variable.

Common logarithm Logarithm of base 10.

Complementary event The probability that an event will not happen. The probability of a complementary event may be found as 1 minus the probability of the primary event. If $\overline{A}$ is the complement of event A, then

$$P(\overline{A}) = 1 - P(A)$$

Confounder An extrinsic factor that is associated with a disease outcome and, independent of that association, is also associated with the exposure. Failure to control for a confounder can cause the measured association between exposure and outcome variables to be misleading.

Correlation coefficient A measure of the strength of the linear association between two variables. It assumes that both variables are normally distributed and that a linear association exists between the variables. The correlation coefficient is a scaled range from −1 (perfect negative association) and +1 (perfect positive association). A 0 value means there is no association between the variables. To calculate the correlation coefficient for a sample, we use the following formula:

$$r = \frac{\sum (x_i - \overline{x})(y_i - \overline{y})}{\sqrt{\sum (x_i - \overline{x})^2 \sum (y_i - \overline{y})^2}}$$

Critical value A number from a distribution that we compare with the value obtained from a test statistic to determine whether or not to reject the null hypothesis. We obtain it from the relevant distribution table.

Data Information obtained through observation, experiment, or measurement of a phenomenon of interest; data consists of facts such as numbers, words, observations, measurements, or descriptions.

Degrees of freedom The number of independent pieces of information used to obtain an estimate; the number of independent observations in a sample minus the number of parameters that are estimated from the sample.

Dependency ratio A measure in epidemiology that describes the relationship between those with the potential to be self-supporting and the dependent segments of the population. The formula is

$$\frac{\text{Population} < 15 \text{ and} \geq 65}{\text{Population } 15 - 64} \times 100$$

Determinants The combination of factors (e.g., personal, social, economic, and environmental) that influence the health of individuals and groups.

Descriptive methods Techniques used to describe data; surveys, case studies, developmental studies, correlational studies, etc.

Distribution In epidemiology, "distribution" refers to the frequency and pattern of health-related states or events.

Epidemic curve A graph of the frequency or magnitude of disease across time, showing the course of the health problem. It identifies the most likely time of exposure and is used to formulate hypotheses about the type of disease involved and its mode of transmission.

Epidemiology The study of the distribution and determinants or health-related states or events in human populations and the application of the study to the prevention and control of health problems.

Equation A statement indicating that the values of two mathematical expressions are equal.

Estimate (also called "point estimate") The actual numerical value obtained for an estimator.

Estimator A random variable or a sample statistic that is used to estimate an unknown population parameter.

Event One or more outcomes of an experiment.

Experiment An operation that consists of a number of independent trials (replications of experiments) under stable conditions and results in any one of a set of outcomes; it is an operation that produces observations or measurements. The actual outcome cannot be predicted with certainty.

Exponent A quantity that reflects the power to which a number or expression is raised.

Exposure Data that reflects an environmental contaminant (e.g., toxic chemical), a behavior (e.g., physical activity), or an individual attribute (e.g., age).

Formula A special type of equation frequently used in epidemiology that shows the relationship between different variables.

Functional relationship Each independent (input) variable is paired with exactly one dependent (output) variable; it is distinct from a statistical relationship.

Frequency distribution A tabular summary of a set of data that shows the frequency or number of data items that fall in to each of several distinct classes; a frequency table.

Geographic information system (GIS) A computer technique that combines spatial information with one or more layers of attribute information; an approach for gathering, managing, and analyzing data.

Graph A diagram that shows the relationship between variables, typically of two variables (i.e., a two-dimensional drawing showing a relationship between two sets of information or numbers).

Hypothesis testing This is a procedure based on sample information and probability that is used to test statements regarding a characteristic of one or more populations. There are six steps to hypothesis testing: (1) formulate a statement about the population parameter called the "null hypothesis"; (2) formulate a statement that contradicts the null hypothesis, called the "alternative" or "research hypothesis";

(3) select the sample size and the level of significance for the statistical test; (4) select the appropriate test statistics and identify the degrees of freedom and the critical value; (5) collect the data and calculate the statistic; and (6) reject or fail to reject the null hypothesis.

Incubation period The time between exposure to a pathogen (e.g., virus, bacteria, fungus parasite), chemical, or radiation and the clinical manifestations of the disease.

Index case The first case to come to the attention of the investigators in an epidemiologic study.

Integers (also called whole numbers) The numbers 0, 1, −1, 2, −2, …, and so on.

Irrational number Number that cannot be expressed as the ratio of two integers.

Level of confidence This applies when the researcher says that the hypotheses will be accepted only if we can have $(1 - \alpha) \times 100$ confidence that the result actually represents the truth.

Level of significance This is the probability of a Type I error, denoted by the Greek letter alpha (α). It is typically set at 0.05, as determined by the investigator.

Likert scale Rating scale that generally involves an odd number of choices (usually 1–5 or 7), ranging from least to most.

Logarithm A quantity that represents the power that a fixed number (also called the "base") is raised to produce a specific number.

Logistic regression A regression technique that is necessary if the outcome variable is dichotomous (two levels) rather than numerical. Logistic regression is commonly used in epidemiology because many of the outcome measures considered involve nominally scaled data.

Measures of central location The commonly used measures of central tendency are the arithmetic mean (average of a set of numbers), median (middle value), and mode (most frequent value). Other measures of central tendency are the midrange (sum of the lowest and highest values divided by 2) and geometric mean (central number in a geometric progression; nth root of the product of n numbers).

Measures of spread Two common measures of spread are the range (difference between the lowest and highest values) and standard deviation (square root of the average of the squared differences from the mean).

Mediator Intermediate in the causal connection between the exposure and outcome variables.

Medical geography An area of health research that studies how locale and climate influence health-related states or events.

Moderator A variable that affects the strength of the relationship between an exposure and outcome variable. The effect of a moderating variable is represented statistically as an interaction.

Natural logarithm Logarithm of base *e*.

Null hypothesis Some postulated belief about the population; it is what is currently believed, or the status quo. It is a formal basis for a statistical test.

Number line Every real number has a unique point on a number line. For any real number, those to the right of 0 on the number line are positive numbers (all numbers *a* with $a > 0$), and all numbers to the left of 0 on the number line are negative numbers (all numbers *b* with $b < 0$). Nonnegative numbers are all numbers *a* with $a \geq 0$.

Numbers Arithmetic values used in counting, making calculations, identifying subjects, and showing the position in a series.

Objective probability The likelihood of the outcome of any event based on repeated random experiments or measurements rather than on subjective assessment.

One-sided test In hypothesis testing, we evaluate whether a parameter is either significantly greater than or less than a given value—not both.

p-value The probability that an effect that is as large or larger than that observed in a particular study could have occurred by chance alone, given that the null hypothesis is true.

Parameter A summary measure of a characteristic from the population.

Person Characteristics include inherent traits (e.g., age, gender, race/ethnicity), activities (e.g., occupation, leisure, use of medications, education, marriage, family), and conditions (e.g., access to health care, clean water, goodhousing conditions; sanitation). The reason certain health-related states or events occur among some people but not others may provide insight into what may be causing a health problem.

Place Areas such as residence, birthplace, place of employment, school district, hospital unit, country, county, census tract, street address, map coordinates, and so on. The concentration of cases may be identified by place and may provide insight when events occur in some places but not others.

Point estimate (also called "estimate") A single numerical value obtained as an estimate of a parameter.

Poisson regression A form of regression analysis in which we model count or rate data. The dependent variable is assumed to have a Poisson distribution.

Proportion A part or amount in relation to a whole.

Rate A proportion that reflects the change in the frequency of one quantity relative to the change in another quantity; a proportion with an added dimension of time.

Ratio A part divided by another part. It is the number of observations with the characteristic of interest divided by the number without the characteristic of interest.

Rational numbers Consist of all fractions of the ratio or quotient of two integers (a/b), where *a* and *b* are integers and $b \neq 0$. Some real numbers are not rational numbers.

Real numbers Values that represent quantities on a number line.

Regression analysis A process of estimating the relationship between a dependent variable and one or more independent variables. A primary strength of this technique is that it can be used to estimate the association between variables that are generally not perfectly associated. The method is also useful for assessing associations between variables while controlling for the confounding influence of other variables.

Relative frequency The frequency of a given category divided by the total number of observations; the frequency in a given category compared with the total of all categories.

Residual An estimate of the random population error; $e_i = y_i - \hat{y}_i$.

Risk factors Attributes, characteristics, behaviors, or exposures associated with the increased production of an adverse health-related state or event.

Sample A subset of items selected from a population.

Sample space The set of all possible outcomes of an experiment.

Sampling frame A unique identifying number that is required for probabilistic sampling, data linkage, and confidentiality; the actual set of units from which a sample will be drawn.

Simple linear regression Involves an equation with one explanatory variable. This method fits a linear line to the data that minimizes the squared deviations of each point from the estimated straight line. The equation is

$$Y = \beta_0 + \beta_1 X + \epsilon$$

Simple random sample A sample that is selected from a finite population in such a way that all samples of the same size have the same probability of being chosen.

Spatial data Describes location. There are four types of spatial data: (1) continuous (e.g., elevation, ultraviolet exposure, precipitation) areas (unbounded: radon gas, forests, land use; bounded: city, county, state, and health boundaries); (2) moving (e.g., mosquito areas, air masses, ozone gas); (3) networks (e.g., roads, rivers, power lines); and points (fixed, such as wells, addresses, street lights; or moving, such as cars, airplanes, animals).

Spearman rank correlation coefficient A measure of association between the ranking of two variables.

Standardized test statistic This is used to determine whether there is sufficient evidence from a sample to reject the null hypothesis. The test statistic compares results from a sample with a hypothesized value. The general formula for a standardized test statistic is

$$\frac{\text{Statistic} - \text{Parameter}}{\text{Standard deviation or Standard error}}$$

Statistical modeling In epidemiology, this involves the activity of translating a real public health problem into mathematics for subsequent analysis. Statistical models describe patterns of association and interactions in data. These models allow us to evaluate variables that predict or explain the outcome variable of interest and whether variables modify this relationship.

Statistic A summary measure based on sample data.

Statistical relationship Unlike a functional relationship, which associates an input variable with an output variable, a statistical relationship is not a perfect one; it is a combination of deterministic and random relationships. All observations do not generally fall on the curve of relationship. Instead, there is a scattering of points around the line conveying the statistical relationship.

Stratified random sample (also sometimes called "proportional" or "quota" random sampling) A sampling approach that involves dividing the population into non-overlapping subgroups (strata), $N_1 + N_2 + \cdots + N_i = N$ and then taking a simple random sample of $f = n/N$ in each subgroup. Stratified random sampling ensures that key subgroups of the population are represented, thus allowing you to be able to say something about these groups in your analysis. It also provides more statistical precision than simple random sampling if the strata are homogeneous.

Subjective probability The personal notion of probability, based on opinion and past experience rather than on formal calculations. It is influenced by personal judgment as to whether a given event will occur.

Systematic sample One where every kth item is selected. Systematic sampling should only be used when a cyclic repetition is not inherent in the sampling frame.

t-distribution A theoretical probability distribution, which is symmetric and bell-shaped and has a mean of 0. It is similar to the standard normal distribution, except it has more area in the tails and the middle is not as high.

t-score Similar to a z-score, but a sample-based standard deviation is used in the conversion.

Time Includes chronological events, step-by-step occurrences, chains of events tied to time, and the time distribution of the onset of cases, all of which can provide insight into what may be causing a health problem.

Two-tailed test In hypothesis testing, we evaluate whether a parameter is both significantly greater than or less than a given value.

Type I error Rejection of the null hypothesis when it is true.

Type II error Failure to reject the null hypothesis when it is false.

Variable A condition, factor, or trait that varies from one observation to the next, may be measured or categorized, and can take on a specified set of values. It represents a number we do not know yet, as opposed to a fixed number.

z-distribution A normal distribution where the mean is equal to 0 and the standard deviation is equal to 1. It is also called the "standard normal distribution."

z-score A number that indicates how many standard deviations an element is from the mean.

Index